AGAINST
THE WIND

AN IRONWOMAN'S RACE FOR
HER FAMILY'S SURVIVAL

LEE DIPIETRO

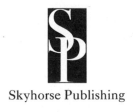

Skyhorse Publishing

Skyhorse Publishing books may be purchased in bulk at special discounts for sales promotion, corporate gifts, fund-raising, or educational purposes. Special editions can also be created to specifications. For details, contact the Special Sales Department, Skyhorse Publishing, 307 West 36th Street, 11th Floor, New York, NY 10018 or info@skyhorsepublishing.com.

Skyhorse® and Skyhorse Publishing® are registered trademarks of Skyhorse Publishing, Inc.®, a Delaware corporation.

Visit our website at www.skyhorsepublishing.com.

10 9 8 7 6 5 4 3 2 1

Library of Congress Cataloging-in-Publication Data is available on file.

Cover design by Rain Saukas
Cover photo credit: Lee DiPietro

Print ISBN: 978-1-63450-452-2
Ebook ISBN: 978-1-63450-470-6

Printed in the United States of America

Dedication

To my husband, Lee,
and our two sons, Tim and Cryder,
for their love, their trust,
and their courage

Contents

Prologue

On a cold and dark February morning in 2010, my husband and I drove from our home about twenty minutes north of Baltimore to the massive Johns Hopkins Hospital. We had allowed ourselves plenty of time just in case morning rush hour had begun. In all the years we'd lived so nearby, I'd never been to the Hopkins medical center, though I'd certainly heard of its excellent reputation and felt lucky to have it in our backyard, particularly now. We rode in silence on the highway towards the city, both of us nervous and anxious to have answers to our questions. The what-ifs were haunting me, but I kept those fears to myself.

Reaching our exit and turning left towards Hopkins, we navigated our way through a rough part of the city where I'd never been. I stared out my window and watched the life of the inner city unfold. A few minutes later, Lee wound the car up to the fifth floor of the crowded concrete garage and parked; then we trudged down five flights of stairs to a long brick walkway that led us to a large complex of buildings. Finally, we entered the main level of the Hopkins Outpatient Center, which was just as crowded as the garage, though with people rather than cars.

The two-story foyer is intimidating—cold glass and steel—and I felt a chill run through my body. I reached for Lee's hand, wanting to feel the warmth of his skin as we threaded our way between throngs of people. At the reception desk, visitors' bands were fastened around our wrists; then, along with everyone else, we shuffled through the turnstile. In the elevator Lee and I clasped hands, though I'm not sure who was reassuring whom. Most people kept their eyes focused ahead, not bothering to share a good morning smile. The doors opened onto the third floor, and we walked down a portrait-lined corridor to the office of a surgeon who held our future in his hands.

His secretary greeted us and we introduced ourselves, apologizing for being a little early. She ushered us through a door to our right.

The doctor rose from his desk to greet us as we stepped through his doorway and invited us to sit at a small conference table in the middle of the room. He was as I had imagined: somewhere in his late fifties, graying hair, reading glasses perched on his nose, and a friendly demeanor. He smiled as he commented on how unusual it was for my husband and me to have the same first names—Lee and Lee. We were used to this—we'd heard the remark often in the more than thirty years that we had been together. Then the doctor excused himself for a minute and returned to his desk to finish answering an email.

Nervously lost in our own thoughts, Lee and I scanned the documents on the walls and photos on the shelves. I wanted to say something to break the silence, make us relax a little, but I couldn't think of anything so I again reached for Lee's hand, this time under the table. His palms were damp like mine. Finally, the doctor turned from his computer and joined us, sitting at the head of the table to my left. Lee sat at my right. We were ready to begin a difficult conversation.

But it didn't go the way I had imagined.

He apologized again for tending to his emails. Then, looking inquisitively at me over the top of his reading glasses, he said: "So I hear you are quite an accomplished runner and triathlete?" He asked me about my marathons and seemed especially impressed that I had competed in several Ironman triathlons in Hawaii. I was surprised he knew all this and wondered why.

I had, indeed, been running for nearly thirty years, winning a number of races and moving up the running echelon into elite status. I had started running in my mid-twenties, and now at fifty-one I still ran competitively. But it was my triathlon experience, particularly in the Ironman, that amazed people. Just what, they strove to understand, drives a person to tackle such a test of endurance, both physical and mental? To swim 2.4 miles, then sprint out of the water to bike for 112 miles, followed by a full marathon of 26.2 miles, all in the same day and without stopping. And not just completing these distances but racing them. Insanity? Surely a bit. Persistence? Yes. Passion, ambition, and dedication? Definitely. The Ironman triathlon is a challenge to see just what your body can do when pushed to extremes. It tests you both physically and mentally, and it lets you know the stuff you are made of. Competing in the race is an incredible accomplishment. Succeed in an Ironman and you feel you can face any trial.

To the doctor I wanted to say, "I am many things, a mother, a wife, a sister, and a daughter. But being a runner and triathlete has made me who I am." Then, returning his curious gaze, I finally answered him. "Yes, Dr. Frassica, I am a runner and a triathlete."

His smile faded as he picked up his pen to make some notes and sketch several diagrams on a white pad of paper. Staring at the drawings, I clutched Lee's hand as the doctor began to explain the battle that lay ahead for us.

1

Running: The Beginning

There was a time in my life, in my mid-thirties to mid-forties, that I was somewhat famous. Not as a celebrity but as a world-class long-distance runner and professional triathlete. I was a local hero not only to runners but to those who saw me run everywhere and every day, in rain, snow, sleet, or heat waves. I was always there, like the mailman. You could count on that. And nationally, I made a name for myself amongst the endurance athletes—runners, triathletes, and duathletes—and their followers, some that I raced against and some that knew of my reputation. I was not only a mom of two young sons and a wife, I had another identity, one that gave me confidence and fed my appetite to be strong and stand out. I became like Clark Kent and Superman; put on my running gear and I transformed from ordinary mom and wife to Superwoman. I was ready to tackle anything that challenged me or my family.

At the peak of my career at age thirty-nine, I placed sixth in the Ironman World Championship in Hawaii, ranking me among the top female Ironman triathletes in the world. And in my forties I was ranked among the top masters long-distance runners in the country. My passion for endurance sports has led me on a path I never would have imagined; a path that was my destiny for a reason. But this was a life that had not been planned since childhood, it was one I fell into it from a simple suggestion.

∿ ∿ ∿

"Come run with me," challenged my sister Kitty, "in the Boston Marathon!"

I was twenty-six, had never run more than four miles at a time, despite years or organized sports, and had no idea how to run the 26.2 miles of a marathon. Her suggestion surprised me, but I was tempted. After all, I had been running a few miles several times a week when I could find the time, trying to keep myself in shape.

"Come on," she said, "Brewster is running too, and it would be fun!"

Fun? I thought. Could be, but the idea was also daunting. Kitty was only asking me to join her at the sixteen-mile mark to help her finish. Could I really run ten miles, in Boston, on that famous, most prestigious marathon course?

Kitty lived in Boston and had been running in the marathon for several years. I'd been a big Boston Marathon fan during my college days attending Boston University, but only as a spectator. Every Patriot's Day in April, I had joined the thousands of waving, screaming onlookers who cheered the runners along their route from Hopkinton into downtown Boston. I'd often watched with envy, blending in with the mass of people on the sidelines, and could only imagine what it would feel like to run a marathon with so many people cheering you on.

Kitty was going to run that year as she always did, as a bandit. There is a strict qualifying time for runners to compete in Boston, but back then, in 1985, unregistered participants were allowed to run. These runners didn't need to qualify to run, were not awarded finisher's medals, couldn't win prizes, and had to start way at the back of the fifteen-thousand-plus registered runners. But these bandits would run the same streets, test themselves in the same way, and feel the same exhilaration as the real Boston Marathoners. This was my chance to see what it felt like from the other side, as a runner.

"I'm game!" I told Kitty enthusiastically.

There was, of course, work to be done in the four months I had to train. I had no idea how to prepare to run ten miles, though I had always been athletic and competitive. Even as a child I had been very successful in sports, playing tennis and being the big winner on the summer swim team. I realize now that having been the middle child of five girls meant I had to find a way to stand out and get noticed, especially by my parents. And I was a much better athlete than student. I felt so proud to come home and tell my parents I had won something and to have them give me the praise I longed for. This need only grew after my parents' divorce. It was then, in middle school and high school, that I joined the field hockey, basketball, and lacrosse teams.

My need to compete continued into college where I played on the lacrosse team at Boston University. I suppose my first exposure to running started then as I'd scramble at the beginning of January, after a long fall of inactivity, to get in shape for the spring lacrosse season with short one- to two-mile runs around the reservoir. In the beginning, those runs were awful. I felt fifteen pounds overweight, even though I wasn't, and my lungs burned with each desperate gasp for air, while my feet hit heavily on the ground. The only way to get in shape meant withstanding the pain and committing myself to a grueling routine. After a few weeks of sore muscles and leaden feet, I found myself looking forward to my vigorous daily runs. My body began to respond to my steps with a feeling of exuberance as I seemingly sprang off the ground with each foot strike. But now, to train for a marathon, I would have to go through that pain again. I reminded myself of that.

Right after college, Lee and I married and moved to the village of Sea Cliff on the north shore of Long Island. I had only done a little running since graduating from college. In the first two years of our marriage and before the birth of our children, my husband and I had become avid tennis players, making time on weekends to get some exercise while socializing with friends. But we couldn't carve out enough time during the week to play as much tennis as I wanted, and I found that taking off for a mile or two whenever I could, eased the tension from the long commute to my job at a decorator's fabric house in Manhattan.

None of that, however, prepared me for my first few runs to get in shape for the ten miles I would run in the Boston Marathon. Initially, the runs were torture, and I dreaded them—my legs felt like lead, I couldn't catch my breath, and the soreness in my legs seemed to persist for days. And then came the increases in mileage; more torture! Those were struggles—both enduring the pain and completing the mileage. At the end of the day, I usually had little energy left, but I forced myself to continue with my plan.

Finding the time to get in shape became another challenge. Not only was I a new mother taking care of our eighteen-month-old son, Tim, but I also worked part-time. And Lee, though very supportive, had to spend long hours building his insurance business. So, on weekdays, I had to fit in runs when I could. On occasion, Lee came home early enough for me to sneak in a run and for him to get time alone with his son. Lucky for both of us, Tim was a very good baby, and my mother, who lived nearby, also took turns babysitting to support my newfound habit.

Still, despite having been a lacrosse player in college and knowing that the only way to get in shape was by committing to a grueling routine, I knew nothing about training for a long distance run. Initially, I trained by taking Kitty's suggestion of simply logging three miles each day. That was at the beginning. Then, over the course of the next three months, she encouraged me to increase the distance every couple of weeks until my longest run of eight miles. You can't increase too quickly because your body needs time to adapt to the mileage by getting stronger and fitter.

But after a few weeks, dressed in my own running gear and hair tugged back in a ponytail, I began to feel re-energized (after the endorphins kicked in), and by the end of each run I noticed I felt stronger and still had energy left to cope with my mom and wife duties.

Not long after that, my body began to change—I lost the baby fat I'd gained with my first pregnancy, saw new muscles, and learned to love the freedom I felt when running. It became the time, carved out of each day, when I could indulge in whatever thoughts I wanted, and did not have to respond to anyone else's needs, including my baby's demands, which could be constant. In fact, running quickly became an addiction. I often found myself pacing as the hour approached when Lee would return from work, watching out the window with Tim in my arms. When Lee finally did arrive, I'd dash out the door to get my fix. A half hour later, I'd return home tired but also refreshed and with a sense of pride. I definitely felt stronger, and the confidence I'd had as a young athlete was returning.

Several weeks before the marathon, Kitty came down to Long Island to join me at my mother and stepfather's house for a training run. She had planned an eight-mile loop to test my readiness, and I was pumped and full of energy as we started to stretch our quads and hamstrings in the driveway. Mom stood with us, watching over Tim as he gleefully mimicked our stretching technique.

Kitty and I took off, and I kept pace as she easily chatted about the course we would run and the rush we'd get from the energetic crowds. I couldn't wait, and I discovered that having someone to talk to while running made the time go by so much faster. Before I knew it, we'd almost arrived home. I still felt strong and knew I was now ready to run Boston.

As we ran up the last hill and rounded the corner to our driveway, we spotted Mom and Tim in the field next to her house, waiting for us. Tim spotted us too and screeched with excitement, which acted like a shot of adrenalin. With a spurt of energy, I sped through the field toward my son. Then, with a last surge of effort, I collapsed on the ground with him and we rolled onto our backs as he squealed with joy. In years to come and at the countless races I ran, I would hear those shouts of encouragement many times from my family, and they always gave me an instant charge. They lifted me up and energized me.

When race day arrived, I awoke early and impatient. Too nervous to eat or sit, I wandered around the house waiting to leave. Kitty had left much earlier to make the thirty-minute drive to the start in Hopkinton. Brewster, our brother, arrived at Kitty's house mid-morning to wait with me and strategize our run. Mom, our biggest fan and supporter, had decided to come up and watch us all. Unfortunately, Lee had to stay home with Tim, who was a little too young to make the trip.

Mom drove Brewster and me to the sixteen-mile mark, where we then waited and cheered others on, hoping that Kitty's predicted time to reach this spot would be accurate. Hundreds and thousands of runners passed, young and old, fit and not. Some appeared energetic, springing from step to step, while others were practically doubled over, staring at the ground in front of them as if in a trance. Some waved at the crowd, encouraging their cheers, and others focused on the road ahead.

Finally, we spotted Kitty, and my heart began to race. It was time to go. Brewster and I jumped in alongside her, as if we were her bodyguards. I felt the urge to sprint ahead, but, as if restraining a horse with reins, I pulled myself back. We were there to run Kitty to the finish, not leave her behind. She had, after all, already run sixteen miles.

As we approached the famed three-mile climb at Heartbreak Hill, at mile seventeen, I could hear the rambunctious spectators encouraging the runners up the start of that long ascent. The crowds were incredible; I had never experienced anything like it. Yes, there had been spectators at my lacrosse games in college, but the fans here exuded as much energy on the sidelines as the marathoners did on the roads. And they were so close to the runners, creating a tunnel along the street for us to run through. Although I was amongst hundreds of other runners, I felt as though the people lining the route were all cheering for only me!

When we ran through Kenmore Square, with only about a mile to go, the three of us began to speed up, weaving through the masses of runners, registered as well as bandits. The cheers from the crowds elevated our spirits as well as our pace. We rounded the last corner onto Boylston Street and saw the finish line several long blocks away, but the excitement of finishing seemed to quicken our steps. The roar of the crowd was deafening, and with our ears buzzing, the three of us clasped hands and raised them over our heads as we crossed the finish line together. I was on cloud nine!

Kitty, whose seemingly boundless energy after running 26.2 miles had truly impressed me, looked as if she could still run some more. Her satisfied and proud smile stretched across her face as wide as mine. I knew immediately that I would do this again. If all these people could run a marathon, then so could I. But next time I would run the full 26.2 miles.

In the hours after the marathon, as Kitty, Brewster, and I relived the race, I was still bursting with excitement and wondered if I could actually run a full marathon. It only took a little coaxing from Kitty before I firmed my decision to run my own marathon. Kitty suggested I tackle the New York Marathon in November. Why not start big?

On the way home to my family in Sea Cliff, the memory of running those miles in Boston stayed with me. The crowds had lured me into a high I hadn't felt since scoring the winning goal in a high-stakes lacrosse game. I wanted that feeling again. My goal was set. I had six months to train.

2

November 2009

We felt fortunate to have both sons with us at Thanksgiving in 2009, as Tim now worked full-time in New York City, in the insurance business like his father, and Cryder, a senior at the University of North Carolina in Chapel Hill, was facing his final season as a star lacrosse player.

By the time the four of us arrived in Delray Beach, Florida, to spend Thanksgiving (a tradition we'd begun a few years earlier) I had run in countless races, including marathons, triathlons, and several Ironmans, winning some, placing in others, and losing a few I thought I should have won. I was also in Delray to train for the Palm Beach Marathon, held during the first week in December, to redeem myself after a disappointing race a month earlier.

I had won the Palm Beach Marathon (among the women) in 2008, when I was fifty years old. It was an incredible thrill to finally win a big marathon, particularly at my age! But the previous October I had fared badly in the Baltimore Marathon. I felt I was in shape to run a 2-hour, 55-minute race but my body thought differently. I was not light on my feet at the midway point, and the fatigue came much too early in the race. I struggled to keep my pace for the last eight miles. I ran a 3:02:16, a very respectable time but not up to my standards, and so I felt defeated and disappointed, particularly with my sixteenth overall finish and third place masters finish. Palm Beach would be my chance to turn that disappointment around, as I had done throughout my years of racing; go back to the drawing board, figure out what went wrong, regroup, and try again. By the time we arrived in Delray, I had two weeks before the race which I hoped was enough time to acclimate to the warmer temperatures.

∾ ∾ ∾

As a child I'd weathered some tough times, especially the year my parents divorced in 1966, when I was only eight, and when many still considered the breakup of a marriage taboo and rather shameful. But nothing compared to the storm that was brewing as we ate our Thanksgiving dinner in 2009, when I was fifty-one and thinking life was becoming simpler again.

All I can say is that little prepares you for the worst year of your life, though having been an Ironwoman and a runner can help. My years of training and racing taught me valuable lessons about myself and life and overcoming obstacles I thought impossible to beat. Ultimately, surviving this ordeal boiled down to my runner's determination: I simply had to win the toughest race of my life.

∾ ∾ ∾

Before I get to the events surrounding Thanksgiving, something had happened a couple of weeks earlier, before we arrived in Delray, and bothersome thoughts had settled into my subconscious, periodically surfacing and making me wonder if something was wrong with Lee.

In early November, Tim, Lee, and I went to Charleston, South Carolina, for the first wedding of one of Tim's high school "gang." All the boys had gathered there, and celebration filled the weekend— parties, dining, dancing. On Sunday morning after all the festivities had ended, I left our hotel room for my usual morning run while Lee promised to follow with his morning walk. It had been a late night on Saturday but we needed to sweat a little poison out of our systems. I struggled through my run and came back to find Lee still lounging and watching TV, claiming his leg was bothering him and that he didn't feel well. I gave him one of my questioning looks and said, "Wouldn't be due to trying to keep up with the boys, or the rock-star dancing you did last night, would it?" We laughed it off and packed our bags to head home.

By the time we got to the airport that afternoon, though, Lee felt worse and was clearly not looking his best. Our flight took us into Philadelphia from where we planned to drive home to Baltimore. We had separate seats on the plane, and when we reunited in Philadelphia, Lee said he still felt awful and now thought he had a fever. He didn't think he could drive.

I'd been married to Lee for almost thirty years and had started dating him in college, so I had seen him through a number of hangovers and illnesses, and he wasn't handling this one well at all, whatever it was. I drove the hour and a half home while he slept. We figured he had picked up some kind of bug, and I felt sorry for him. The next morning, he awoke with a slight cough but said he felt much better. As we thought: just a twenty-four-hour bug.

Over the next few days when Lee came home in the evening from his insurance business, dragging a bit and coughing occasionally, I still didn't think much of it. It wasn't unusual for him when he felt poorly to just sit on the sofa looking like he'd lost his best friend while he sniffled and coughed and held tight to the TV remote, channel surfing. I would roll my eyes. I cared, but, honestly, it was just a cold.

I had hoped that he'd be over his illness by the time the family arrived in Delray Beach, but instead Lee seemed less energetic and unusually moody. I couldn't figure out what was nagging him, and he wasn't saying. He typically kept such things to himself. All the years we had been together, I had tried to encourage him to share his feelings, as I did. I am one to speak my mind. But Lee still kept some things private until something made them surface. I learned to be patient, at least most of the time.

~ ~ ~

On the Saturday after Thanksgiving we had a gorgeous beach day. After lunch, Tim rented a paddleboard, while Cryder patiently waited to join his older brother in the ocean with his surf-board. I watched them, thinking about how different two children from the same family can be. Tim was our risk taker and thrill seeker, while Cryder took a more cautious approach. Even as a young boy, Tim had absolutely no fear of sharks, in contrast to Cryder. If Tim saw a pod of dolphins swimming a hundred yards out, he'd dash into the water with his bogey board, paddle out to where he'd seen them, and wait until they surfaced again. But not Cryder; he would wait on the shoreline, watching Tim and surely questioning his fearlessness.

On this day, I saw Lee walk down to the edge of the beach, joining Cryder as Tim paddled toward them. I remember the next moment vividly: Lee and Cryder stood together, not far from our beach chairs, while I fidgeted with my camera, ready to play my usual role as photographer.

My cell phone rang. I tried to escape notice that I was breaking the no-cell-phones-on-the-beach rule by smuggling it under the beach umbrella to muffle the sound. In the next instant I heard Brewster's voice saying he had been trying to reach me for two hours. I had obviously not checked my phone for a while.

"Why, what's wrong?" I asked my younger brother.

His next words now echo mournfully in my head: "I called to tell you that Ames is in a better place."

"Ames is what?" What was he saying? Ames, my younger sister?

It took a moment to register what he was trying to tell me about her, and then I knew. I don't remember screaming, but Lee heard me and saw me stagger behind the beach chairs, gasping for breath and enveloped in tears.

I'm not sure how long Brewster talked to me, as time seemed to swim away while I tried to control myself. He talked to calm me down, as only Brewster can do. He reminded me how much Ames had been struggling and how desperate she'd been. Her struggles were now over, he said, and she was at peace. While that should have been a comfort, it was hard to accept.

On the crowded beach, people were camped all around our cabana and chairs. I tried to stay somewhat hidden, but I am sure others heard and saw my outburst. Lee frequently looked to see if I was OK. He and Cryder were obviously concerned but trying not to draw attention to my conversation. When I finally got off the phone, Lee was there in an instant, throwing his arms around me.

I couldn't stop crying. "It's Ames," I said, and he knew.

Lee adored Ames. He had known her since she was fifteen. She had a terrific sense of humor and took great pleasure in finding ways to poke fun at Lee, something he loved and always welcomed. Her suicide shocked and devastated him, as it did me. We sought comfort in each other's arms.

Cryder cast several nervous glances at us as he stood at the edge of the water still waiting for Tim. After a few minutes, I sent Lee to tell him what had happened. Cryder tensed as he listened, then immediately came to me. "I'm so sorry, Mom," he said, and we hugged and shed more tears. Both of the boys knew of Ames's problems with alcohol and depression, and they were keenly aware of the close-knit sisterhood that existed between all of us sisters. Cryder paddled out on his surfboard to tell Tim. I saw Tim's head drop, and then he looked over at me standing on the beach with Lee's arms around me. He paddled in quickly, and like his father and brother before him, he wrapped his big arms around me, while tears slipped down his cheeks.

My strong, loving men surrounded me that afternoon and tried to absorb some of my pain. We stayed on the beach, with the boys riding the waves, and all of us talking about Ames. It was the perfect place to be. Ames, the beachgoer and sun-worshipper, loved to show off her deep tan. That night at dinner I announced that I still planned to run the marathon the following Sunday, but now I would run it for Ames. I'd pin her name to my back and run her to a better place.

∼ ∼ ∼

Training for the Palm Beach Marathon was quite different from training for my first-ever marathon in New York in 1985. At that time, though I'd run ten miles with Kitty in Boston, I still had no idea how to prepare for a full marathon. I didn't have the ease of Googling "training for a marathon" in those days, nor did I know many runners, other than my sister, whose brains I could pick. I had been encouraged, however, after noticing the variety of shapes and sizes of participants while both watching and running in that race, not to mention the span of age groups, which also impressed me. People as young as their late teens and as old as their eighties ran in the marathon. There were short, tiny, skinny runners, heavy runners, tall and lanky runners who looked unbelievably fit, as well as those who looked like they had just rolled off the sofa. So, even without access to other marathon runners besides Kitty, I figured that if all these people could train to run a marathon, then, with my athletic background and my drive to compete, I should have no trouble with this challenge.

Still, finding the time to learn and train became another issue. Working part-time and doing my best as a mother and wife, it became quite a juggling act to fit in running, relying on my mother and husband to babysit. As far as I knew, you just ran your few miles and returned home, which I did about four times a week. My sister helped me, sharing her training routine and letting me know I had to run at least half the distance or more by October, a few times before the race in November. At my sister's advice, I knew my goal was to work up to running at least fourteen to sixteen miles a few times before the race in November.

So between May and September I increased my mileage every few weeks. When I ran my longest run of about sixteen miles several weeks before the marathon, I felt as if I had been running for days by the time I got home. It was a long way, but I figured that if I could run for sixteen miles, another ten couldn't be that difficult. Wrong assumption.

Although running had become very popular in the eighties, getting a spot in the New York Marathon in 1985 was not as difficult as it is now. That year would be my first race ever with my own number pinned to my chest. On race day, the Sunday before Halloween, I again felt restless. All runners had to be dropped off at the start of the race on the west side of the Verrazano Bridge. Thousands of people gathered there, wandering about or claiming a spot to sit and wait. The lines for the Porta Potties snaked everywhere. It looked like a tent city, with people wrapped in blankets and their bags of supplies at their feet.

I had come to the race with a group of friends—all male racing veterans—and we waited together. They had run this marathon before and knew the routine, which they happily passed on to me. They told me, for instance, to make sure that when I got to the finish line that I didn't stop—I had to keep moving until I got to the shoots or I would get in the way of the other finishers. "Shoots?" They looked at me, stunned. (Well, it *was* my first race.) The shoots, they explained, were the roped-off alleys that a finisher continued through to get a medal and foil blanket. This was totally new to me. Bandits were not allowed through the shoots at the Boston Marathon, but as a registered runner in New York I would be, so this time I would be awarded my first finisher's medal.

About a half hour before the gun went off, the guys pulled me along with them through the packs of runners, positioning us in our starting corrals among the other jittery runners. Our starting positions were determined by the finish times we had predicted when registering for the race, and so we now looked for those times on signs posted at intervals along the starting line. My mouth was dry and my stomach unsettled as I readied to run. With minutes to go before the start, the national anthem played, and then I heard the starting gunshot. I could see in the distance ahead the crowds of runners bobbing up and down as if running in place. The wave of bobbing moved back toward me, and then in one movement the runners around me lurched forward and suddenly we were off and headed across the Verrazano Bridge. I felt as though I were being pulled along by the energy of my fellow runners, at the same time experiencing enormous relief as my nervous stomach calmed for the long run ahead.

When I hit the Bronx, though, about eighteen miles into the race, my legs suddenly felt like cement. Several miles before that I'd begun to slow down, but I kept telling myself, "Of course, you are tired, but keep running." Other runners had told me about "hitting the wall." In a marathon, that tends to happen around eighteen miles. That wall was definitely in my path and getting larger.

I'd already passed many runners who had slowed to a walk, but even as I trudged along, I still passed runners who'd started before me. Except now I was feeling the pain and struggling with each step. *Be tough, be strong, you can do this*, I urged myself forward. *Don't give up*. My running became a slow jog with constant breaks of walking. Pain seared through my legs with each step, but I continued moving forward. I knew my husband and my mother were waiting for me at the finish line in Central Park. I made seeing them—pleasing them—my goal. I convinced my body to keep going. Mind over matter.

When I rounded the corner onto Fifth Avenue, approaching the final mile of the race, I felt a surge of energy. And as I finally turned into Central Park and heard my family wildly cheering for me, my legs felt light, almost as if they were no longer there. I ran across the finish line four and a half hours after I started. I felt overwhelmed with emotion. I did it! With some difficulty, I made my legs move again and followed the other runners through the shoots, proudly ducking my head to have one of the volunteers drape my medal over my shoulders. I threaded my way through the masses of runners cloaked in foil blankets to the family reunion area, grabbing bottles of water from volunteers as I walked on.

There, Lee was waiting for me with a huge smile and his fists pumping toward the sky. He wrapped his arms around me, and I finally let myself collapse into him. As we walked back to our hotel together, it took me all of about thirty minutes to forget the pain and quietly decide: I had to do this again. But next time I would be better prepared. I would be stronger and more confident. I wanted to keep running. I wanted to be good at this new sport.

3

The Cushing Girls minus One

Preparing for the Palm Beach Marathon in 2009 posed a different kind of challenge. I was grieving and my heart was filled with sadness. Running was my place to be alone, to make sense of things. So, every run, I inevitably thought of Ames, of my childhood, my other sisters. I recalled how close we had been and all the challenges we'd faced together, especially after our parents' divorce.

We were the Cushing Girls, five of us born within five years in the late 1950s. We lived comfortably on the north shore of Long Island—not privileged, just comfortable. When we were very young and spent our summers on the beach, we were labeled the Five Cushing Mermaids. In our teens, that changed to the Tall Sisters.

For most of our youth, we traveled as a pack. I was the middle child. My two older sisters, Edie and Kitty, were both born in April; the twins, Nini and Ames, came two years after me, in March. We always joked about Mom being in labor for two days with the twins because Dad wanted a boy so badly that neither of the girls wanted to be the first to leave the womb.

As it turned out, I was the tomboy, the son Dad always wanted. I played touch football and was happy when he gave me a plastic Viking warrior sword and shield for Christmas. Kitty was my sidekick. We did everything together as kids (so she got a sword set, too). Edie, the oldest, was the caregiver, our second mother, while the twins stuck together in our family circle. But all five of us, being so close in age, relied on each other for everything: advice, friendship, mischief, and having a scapegoat when we needed to deflect a punishment.

In first grade, I thought we had the perfect family. My father worked hard in the insurance business, and my mother and father appeared to have a happy marriage. But children don't always sense what's going on behind closed doors. And sadly that seemed to be the case with us girls. Our protected world fell apart during the long break between second and third grade. That summer, in 1966, our mother rented a small house on Martha's Vineyard where several of our friends spent part of their vacation each year. My sisters and I were so excited we could hardly wait to get there, but I couldn't understand why we made the trip without my father.

"He'll join us for the weekend," my mother promised.

One night after supper, soon after we arrived in Martha's Vineyard, my mother called us three older girls into her room. Never at a stand-still, I excitedly bounced on her big bed. She told me to stop; she had something important to tell us. Her eyes welled up as she told us that she and our father were separating. I burst into tears and cried hysterically. I didn't understand divorce; all I knew was that it meant the father I adored would no longer live with us. How could this happen? I was Dad's shadow, following him everywhere, crawling into his lap when he read me Winnie-the-Pooh; I was his Tigger and he was my hero. Edie, always the nurturing older sister, tried to comfort me but I refused to be consoled. That summer ended the world we had known. Our father did come for a weekend, but our future had changed and his visit felt bittersweet.

Not much time passed before another man entered our mother's life. This man, Jack, had already been in our lives for some time, in fact. He had been my father's good friend and also the father of one of my best friends. This relationship caused tension, as you can imagine, but as a little girl, I failed to understand adult dynamics.

In the spring of my third grade year, Jack married my mother and suddenly Jack's middle daughter Wendy, my best friend, became my sister. On the last day of school, my sisters and I got off the bus at our new house in Mill Neck, not far from our old one on the north shore of Long Island. It was a gorgeous house, one that Jack had built to fit his new family of five girls while still having enough space for his three daughters when they spent occasional weekends and part of their summer with all of us. When they came we had instant teams for Kick the Can and Red Rover, Red Rover. Though I missed my father terribly, living there should have seemed like a dream; we even had a swimming pool and a children's wing all to ourselves.

However, things were far from perfect. Though Jack could be wonderful to us girls, he also intimidated us. He had a strict set of rules (never leave things laying around, keep your voices down, no rough housing in the house, etc.) and my mother always seemed to be sending us off to the children's wing so we wouldn't impose on her time with him. Each day found us in the same routine. We got off the bus close to five o'clock and walked up the driveway and into the house where our "children's supper" awaited us. We ate dinner, then our mother shooed us off to our rooms to do homework and told us not to return to the kitchen until after she'd finished dinner with Jack. I'm sure she found it difficult to juggle a new husband and her five daughters and did what she thought was best. Still, at times we felt unwanted, and everyone had to adjust.

Jack intimidated my sisters more than me, mostly because I'd already known him for several years. He was mysterious and very cool, a little like James Bond. And perhaps a bit of Ernest Hemingway, as he'd filled one of the rooms in the house, the "game room," with his hunting trophies: a polar bear rug with black claws and a gaping head full of teeth, a lion's pelt, elephant tusks, and the heads of various African animals, such as sables and kudus. This man, who'd shot all these animals, intrigued me, and I wondered what sort of man did that. As with my father, I wormed my way into Jack's heart, showing enthusiasm when he told stories of Africa or his life as a Marine and following in his shadow when I was allowed. Although I idolized this man, in my mind he couldn't fill my father's shoes, and I continued to pine for Dad.

Trips to see our father were sporadic. He had moved into New York City, a place that seemed light years away despite only being about thirty miles and less than an hour's car ride. We spent the occasional weekend with him, and I often counted the days until we could spend a whole week together over spring vacation, or even better, a whole month during summer. However, our fleeting reunions were often difficult; at first, all of us felt awkward, then we'd settle into a comfortable pattern, laughing and at ease again, only to end our visits with tear-filled and agonizing partings. I often cried for days after arriving back in Mill Neck.

While Mom was busy trying to create a new life with our stepfather, we girls—particularly the five of us Cushing girls—relied more and more on each other. Our three stepsisters lived most of the year with their mother in Connecticut. Where we lived, our elementary school ended in ninth grade, and most of the families, including ours, sent their children to boarding school after that.

Before we were sent off, less than two years into the marriage and when I was ten, my half-brother Brewster was born. The little prince, as we liked to call him. Though we loved having a brother, we sometimes felt a little jealous because our parents—my mother and stepfather—accorded superior status to the prince over the five Cushing sisters. As we grew up, particularly during our troublesome teen years, we discovered that "our" rules often didn't apply to him. Even more so, tension arose between Jack and my mother. He could be patient with us up to a point, and then all hell broke loose. At times, his anger frightened us, especially since he was not our real father and we were living in his house. Early on, our mother had instilled in us the need to always be on our best behavior—or else. I now know this wasn't the case, but at the time, I truly feared we might be exiled if we really misbehaved.

～ ～ ～

In the seventies, my sisters and I were testing the limits and trying to find our way. Leaving home for boarding school at the age of fifteen had its trials and tribulations for each of us, particularly when we relied so heavily on each other for guidance and companionship. We did not do so well in boarding school—in fact, my two older sisters were both kicked out their first year away, at which point we began to hear "your children" versus "our children" being tossed about. Ames only made it to her second year before being suspended, and Nini was asked to leave in the fall of her senior year. I managed to make it all the way through—not because I was a Goody-Two-shoes but because I was smart enough not to get caught. I'd learned a few things from my sisters' mistakes.

Those years were tough for all of us. We engaged in a lot of drinking and experimenting with drugs. Luckily for me, playing sports in school held a much greater interest. When home for the holidays, we all tended to gather at the local bars. The drinking age was eighteen then, but it was easy enough to get into the bars at sixteen or younger. We were all a bit shy and tended to stick together. The twins were particularly dependent on each other; one rarely went anywhere without the other. Despite this, our parents sent them to separate boarding schools, and I think that began Ames's struggles.

Moreover, alcoholism ran in our family, and it wasn't long before several of my sisters fell victim to that disease. Ames was the first, at the age of twenty. Shortly after my wedding to Lee everyone recognized that she was struggling. My parents decided then that it would be best to send her off to Minnesota to a program for alcohol abuse. Ames, always pretty stubborn, fought the system for a while, but after a couple of years of the program she became sober and was on her way to a better life. The problem with an alcoholic, however, is that the compulsive behavior can resurface in other areas, even if the drinking ends. Over the years, Ames also battled bulimia and a lack of confidence. When she was still in her twenties, Ames fell in love and married the man of her dreams. They had three wonderful children and a good life together for a long time. It wasn't until the children were much older that Ames started suffering from depression. She fought hard but couldn't seem to shake the vicious grasp it had on her life. She fell back into alcoholism.

Ames and Edie both lived in Newport, Rhode Island, so Edie was there for her, helping to mother her and lift her from her dark moods. Kitty spent summers and weekends in Newport and gave Ames much support, too. Two summers before that phone call on the beach in Delray, I also joined them in Newport for a month after many years of being away. It was the place where we had spent summers with our father years earlier and was still a source of joy and pleasure for all of us. Although Ames and I had kept in touch over the years, we had lost the closeness of our youth.

Living in Baltimore now, I seldom saw her. We would call each other several times a year, and she never missed my birthday, nor I hers. But my life had changed a lot since our youth. I had a family at a young age, and then my involvement in the running and triathlon world kept me busy, putting me on a different path from the ones my sisters were following.

Yet that summer in Newport (2008), I quickly saw how Ames's life had spun out of control. She was depressed, angry, lost, and scared. She loved her children deeply, though, and knew she had to fight to be with her family. That fall, she again entered a rehab institution. It was extremely difficult for everyone, but it had to be done, and she knew it. After her release in the spring of the next year, Ames went home and tried to return to a normal life with her husband and family. But the months away made it difficult to resume life as it had been.

During the summer after her release, in 2009, Ames started to falter again. On the first of August, Lee and I arrived in Newport for a month, our second summer there. The phone rang on the third morning. It was Edie and she sounded terrified. Ames had attempted suicide the night before and was in the hospital. Edie had rushed to her side and had been there much of the night. I felt the breath leave my lungs and a shiver run through my body. Brewster had been warning me for a while that he felt Ames had fallen into a bad place and might kill herself. I didn't believe him. She would never do that—she loved her children too much to leave them.

Ames spent several days in the hospital, and I had long talks with her. I told her we were all there for her and that she had to know she could always turn to any of her sisters for help and support. We would drop everything if she needed us and be at her side in an instant. Through many tears, she said she realized that she had to live to raise her children, and she resolved to fight the demons that possessed her. I believed her.

It was the beginning of November, only a few weeks before her suicide, that I saw her again. We went up to Newport for the night and met Ames at her son's college, where he was playing a soccer game. She seemed like her old self, with her big smile and wonderful belly laugh, an infectious guffaw like no one else's. She appeared happy and in control. Or so it seemed. I have heard from others that someone who is planning suicide is able in the days and even weeks before to put on a front that everything is fine and life is great. The person doesn't want to put others on the alert for what's to come. So it would appear to have been with Ames.

A few months before I saw her at the soccer game, she had moved out of her house into a small cottage, all to herself. It was right around the corner from her children and husband, so she would be close by. She and her husband had decided they needed some time apart to work things out. At the soccer game, she told me how much she loved her cottage and how happy she was. When the game was over, I hugged her good-bye, wished her a happy Thanksgiving with her family, and flew back home to Baltimore. I told her I would be back next summer, and we could spend some time at her favorite place, the beach.

I vowed that I would spend more time with Ames. I felt I could help her get her life back. Ames used to run, and at one point her compulsive behavior turned her into an exercise junkie. She would spend hours on her stationary bike, working up a good sweat. I thought that if I could get her back into running again, she would feel good about herself. Running has been known to help people with depression. It gives them a sense of control over their lives, of empowerment. I believed it would be a way for Ames to take command once again, and I wanted to help her get that chance. Sadly, I was too late.

~ ~ ~

I had the week after Thanksgiving all to myself to continue training for the Palm Beach Marathon and to grieve for my sister. Tim and Cryder had left on Sunday. Lee stayed one more night, and I was glad for his presence as I couldn't stand the quiet. I was so caught up in my own grief that I didn't notice whether Lee seemed ill or not, though probably he suppressed whatever he was feeling in order to be supportive of me. Repeatedly, I found myself dissolving in tears. Why couldn't I have done something to help Ames? Why hadn't I known she was so desperate? She had fooled me into thinking she was happy again. I felt like a terrible sister, too involved in my own life and insensitive to her pain.

After Lee left, I thought a lot about Ames and the good times when we were young and all lived under the same roof. I mostly focused on Ames's happier days. Running on the beach was a good place for me to think. I looked up at the clouds and pictured Ames floating on a white puff of cotton. I tried to imagine shapes that would indicate Ames was up there sending a message. I truly felt she was trying to communicate, trying to tell me she was OK. My other sisters were having similar experiences. We talked often, gaining strength from each other.

I still ran every morning, although not as far as before Thanksgiving because it was time to taper for the marathon. These shorter forty-five- to sixty-minute runs were not, however, feeling as easy as they should. Typically, this was the time I would start to feel more and more energized, like a fenced-in stallion. I had been cutting back on my distance for the past three weeks, and this long taper before the marathon should have shown signs of renewed strength in my legs. But that was not happening. Instead, I felt worn out and heavy on my feet.

Midweek, I felt particularly sluggish as I headed home after an hour-long run. I silently told Ames I might not be able to do this race. Then suddenly, mid-step, I looked down and there, right where my foot was about to land, lay a giant dead iguana. I screamed and somehow leaped over it. Never in the years I'd been running on these roads had I ever encountered a three-foot-long iguana in my tracks, dead or alive. That definitely put some pep in my step. After a minute or so, I burst into laughter as I imagined Ames bent over laughing hysterically, too. I looked up at the clouds and shouted, "That was not funny, Ames!"

The weekend arrived and Lee flew back down from Baltimore to cheer me on. He was still coughing a little and tired but he made no mention of it because of his concern for me. I had won this race the year before, and journalists were quick to report that I'd returned to defend my crown, putting a lot of pressure on me to run fast again. But more than anything I wanted to run well to make Ames proud to have her name on my back.

Both my boys called to wish me luck. I talked to Tim the night before, and Cryder left a voice message I heard when I awoke Sunday morning, telling me he was there in spirit, cheering for me, and knew that I would do well because I was running for Ames. I saved the message and it will always make me think of my sister.

This race concerned me for several reasons. Always before big races, there's a mental checklist I run through. Two big questions headed this list: Did the emotions over the past week take too much out of me? And could I handle the heat? The two questions were related. When I had raced in the Palm Beach Marathon the year before, the heat had been brutal, especially during the last few miles as the temperature rose to more than eighty degrees, much warmer than perfect marathon temperatures hovering in the fifties. And now that I felt more fatigued because of my sorrow, I worried that the heat would be even tougher on me.

Not that I hadn't run in hot and humid races. I'd learned over the years the importance of acclimating your body to the temperatures you'd race in. In the Hawaii Ironman in mid-October, for example, the hot humid summers in Baltimore had helped prepare me, and I would arrive in Hawaii about a week before the race to further acclimate. I also reminded myself about the awful conditions I had raced in at other times and assured myself I could get through the Palm Beach race just as I had survived the Olympic Trials held in Columbia, South Carolina.

❧ ❧ ❧

That day, in February of 2000, they'd expected the temperature to be in the mid-fifties or sixties, but on race day, Mother Nature did not cooperate; instead it rose to eighty-two degrees with high humidity. Perfect! No one was prepared, especially those who'd been training in the cold, as I had been in Baltimore. I had in no way prepared my body to manage that kind of heat, but there was nothing I could do about it. Running in the Olympic trials was a huge honor and I wanted more than anything to perform well. I had driven the course and seen the hills and knew what to expect. It was going to be a tough one. Of course, it should be; it was the Olympic Trials.

As predicted, the temperatures were already soaring early in the morning of race day. I did what I could to prepare and was well hydrated before the race began. I followed my usual routine of stretching and light jogging before the gun would go off. I reminded myself to control what I could control, one of the key lessons I had learned throughout my career. I was so incredibly nervous and honored to be lining up with all these amazingly talented runners. Three of these girls would qualify to run in the Olympics, and I couldn't help but watch the favorites as they followed their prerace routines. I wondered if they were as nervous as me.

When we were all lined up and the national anthem was sung, we stood shoulder to shoulder, bent forward at the waist with fingers ready to press our timers on our watches. I knew I had to hold back in the beginning of the race and not get carried away with the extra energy you felt in the first few miles. With this heat, I knew I had to readjust my pace, slowing it down in order to compensate for temperature and humidity. I positioned myself near a group of girls I knew were planning on running a similar pace. It is helpful to work together, to help each other keep pace, even though you are competing against each other. There will be a time that you will hope to break away and surge away, but in the beginning stages of the race, you try to work together.

The first few miles felt easy and relaxed, just the way I wanted them to feel. By the midway point, I was starting to slow down and felt myself searching for the water stops that would come every mile, though not soon enough. I knew the heat was getting to me and I tried to keep pace with the girls around me, but I was beginning to lose the group I was running with and there was nothing I could do to respond. I knew the signs of fatigue and I could feel my race start to fall apart, but giving up was not an option. I had never dropped out of a race before and now was not the time to start. If I had to hobble and walk, I was going to cross that finish line.

A big contingent of my family came to watch; Lee and our boys, my mother, my sister Edie, my stepsister Wendy and her son Trevor. They had jumped around the course in front of me to several spots along the way and I knew they could sense I was struggling, but their encouragement willed me to continue; I did not want to let them down. My pride was on the line too, as this race was highly publicized and the running world would comb over the results. Running badly would be embarrassing.

I remember approaching the final uphill stretch knowing it would soon level off at the top and then flatten out for the last quarter mile down the main street. The hill looked steeper than I remembered and I just wanted to stop and relieve myself of the agony I was experiencing. "Come on!" I told myself. I took a deep breath, glanced towards the top of the hill, and shuffled my way up with my head bent and shoulders dropped, looking like I was defeated. When I crested the hill, I could hear a familiar voice.

"Mom, Mom, come on! Keep going! Come on, Mom, I will run with you! You can do it!"

It was Cryder who, at thirteen years old, had insisted he run from the finish line, where he was waiting with the rest of the group, down the street to wait for me and run me into the finish. By then, my family knew my predicted finish time had long passed and had become worried. Cryder couldn't sit still and wait for me so he came back to pull me along.

I can't tell you how much that picked me up. I suddenly began to move faster, and as I ran down the road, I could still hear his encouraging voice as he ran behind the crowds lining the street. "You're doing it, Mom. Keep going!" I ran over the finish line, gritting my teeth and ignoring the pain. My time was 2:52:39, which wasn't that bad for a difficult day, but in my eyes far off the sub 2:48 that I wanted to run. As it turned out, it was a difficult day for everyone, and that year only one woman made the qualifying mark at the trials to run in the Olympics.

I tried to console myself with the fact that it was a tough day for everyone, but as is my nature, the only way I could prove to myself that I was the runner I wanted to be was to run again. So in April, two months after that race, I toed the line again in the Boston Marathon and satisfied myself with a 2:47:00 finish. And now I would toe the line in Palm Beach to fix my damaged pride, and run strong for Ames.

The Palm Beach Marathon started at 6 a.m., and we ran the first half hour or so in the dark, during the cooler temperature. If all went well, I would be finished three hours later, before the sun could really wreak havoc. I was surprised at the way my body seemed to come to life as I did my usual pre-race warm-up. I felt springy on my feet, which was a good sign. Maybe I would surprise myself. As we all began to position ourselves at the starting line, I heard Lee's voice calling me; he waved and wished me luck. It gave me a welcoming jolt, and I was ready to go. Lee, my loyal supporter, was there to ride his bike along the course, jumping to spots along the course to cheer me on. It was a huge help to have him there.

As the race unfolded, I found the miles ticking by, and I was still light on my feet. This was what you hope for in a marathon. I was feeling strong and racing as planned. I even led until about mile twenty-two. But then I began to fade, and I struggled to keep my pace. When the second-place woman overtook me, easily passing me, I gave her a thumbs-up and said good job, as we runners do. I wasn't giving up yet, but she looked strong and I owed her the recognition.

It was time to get help. "OK, Ames," I said, "I need some of your angel wings. Get off my back and help me!" Reaching deep within myself once again, and with Ames firmly in my mind, I found the strength I needed for the last four miles as Lee rode his bike in front of me. His encouragement and cheering pushed me over the finish line. My body gave in and my legs burned, and I was instantly relieved. It was over. I came in second overall among the women, and, even more, accomplished my goal of finishing just under 2:55, beating my time from the year before when I won the race. I couldn't have been happier, except of course if I had won! Lee was all smiles and so proud of me for racing under such difficult circumstances, both physically and emotionally.

After he left, and while I was sitting in the park waiting for the awards ceremony, the emotions hit me. I was thinking of Ames and so proud to have carried her with me. My heart ached, and the tears came uncontrollably. I was hoping my dark sunglasses would hide my red swollen eyes when, moments later, I was called to the stage to accept my award. The lump in my throat stung as I shook hands and held up my award. I saved the finisher's medal and the water-stained "Running for Ames" sign to give to her children, wanting them to remember the marathon she and I had run together.

The service for Ames occurred the following weekend in Newport. Lee and I flew back to Baltimore the Monday morning after the race, and I had a few days to gather myself before taking the train to Long Island to be with my mother and brother. From Long Island, Mom, Brewster, and my stepfather Jack and I would drive up to Newport. Lee, who still lacked his usual energy, would fly up and join us in Newport on Friday. When Mom hugged me at the train station on Long Island, I felt the love and comfort that comes from a mother's embrace no matter ones age. I was spent emotionally and physically, and so was she. I could see it in her face, hear it in her voice.

Over the years, my mother and I had become close as friends, particularly after Lee and I moved into the house right next door to her and Jack. Our children were young when we lived in that house, and Mom often lent us a hand. She and I spent time together almost every day, or at least we talked on the phone. We came to know what the other was thinking before the words came out. That day at the train, I could only imagine the pain she felt at losing a child. I was happy to have her in my arms, too. I wanted to take her pain away, to give her some strength.

The next morning, my mother, Jack, Brewster, and I drove up to Newport. It was a blessing to be with Brewster. We, too, are close, and no one is more entertaining. He acted like a rock for all of us and tried to lift everyone's spirits throughout the weekend. We all stayed with my oldest sister, Edie. When we arrived midday, we found Ames's twin, Nini, already there. Although Nini lived hours away in a small town in New York, she and Ames had remained inseparable. They spoke almost daily. But Nini—the youngest (by thirty seconds)—had already had her share of tragedy, which made this so much harder for her. She became the one we all worked hardest to support.

Nini had been married for ten years and was the mother of four children when her youngest daughter started to show signs of underdevelopment. Sienna was a beautiful little girl, but she failed to begin talking or walking when she should. At our mother's insistence, Nini took her to doctors, then specialists. The doctors diagnosed Sienna with a brain-stem disorder that was preventing her from developing properly. It was devastating, but Nini lovingly cared for her very sick child, doing all she could to prolong Sienna's young life.

Then pancreatic cancer struck Nini's husband, Bob. It was a nightmare for their family, for all of us. As he fought hard, their daughter was failing quickly. Sadly, the day after Christmas, fewer than six months after his diagnosis, Bob died. A month later, Sienna died at the tender age of seven. Since then, Nini had been raising her son and two other daughters on her own, eventually becoming a real estate broker in New York.

Now she looked great. I hadn't seen her in several years. After her daughter died, she had gone into a tailspin. She had kept to herself, trying to heal. Her pain had been difficult to watch, but here she was, with the same smile and big open arms.

A group hug, and more tears.

We all busied ourselves in the kitchen, helping Edie get ready for the twenty-five people coming for dinner. As we chopped and cooked, Edie and Nini decided to practice their reading for the service the next day. They were sharing a reading because neither wanted to stand up alone before the gathering. Brewster and I sat still as they composed themselves. Edie read her few lines first. Then, as Nini was about to start her verse, Edie elbowed her to let her know it was her turn. Nini paused mid-sentence and looked aghast at her sister. We all broke up laughing. Through her own laughter, Nini scolded Edie playfully. "I was all in the mood, solemn, focused and ready to read, and you jab me with your elbow!" Although Brewster and I suggested it might help the mood of the church and would be considered typical of the Cushing girls to do something like that at the actual service, we decided not. But the humor that afternoon was a welcome relief.

We were still scrambling with the last-minute rush to get the food ready to serve when the dinner guests arrived. I had not seen Ames's husband or her children since she had died, and I nervously anticipated that moment. They brought with them poster boards covered with wonderful photos of Ames that they'd spent hours putting together to capture her life. The photos brought tears to my eyes as I glanced over all those years and family moments. I so wished she could be standing with us, telling the stories the pictures told. Oh, Ames, what a loss.

Later that evening, when I found a quiet moment with her children, I gave them the crinkled marathon number, the sign I wore declaring that I was "Running for Ames," and the finisher's medal. I was so proud of them as they tried to conceal their breaking hearts.

The service the next day was beautiful and crowded. Nini and Edie remained stoic during their readings, and Ames's three children tried to be brave, as did her husband, who read very touching stories about his life with Ames. With several of my stepsisters there, it felt as if we were a family again. In our college years, when we all got dressed to go out, we used to sing our version of the Sister Sledge song: "We are fam-i-lee . . . I got all my sisters with me." It was one of Ames's favorites, and we laughingly reminisced about our singing and dancing talents. We also, briefly, once again considered lightening up the mood of the service, this time by breaking into this song because it would have given Ames a chuckle.

After the reception, Mom and Jack drove back to Long Island, and my sisters, Brewster, Lee, our sons, and I returned to Edie's for a quiet dinner where we sat around telling more favorite stories about Ames. In hindsight, I recall Lee's downcast mood, but at the time I was more focused on everyone's heartache, not just one person's. Only later did I realize he'd behaved in a more sullen manner than was ordinary for him.

On Sunday morning, I awoke early and snuck down to the kitchen to brew a cup of coffee and enjoy the sunrise. Edie's house faced the beach that Ames loved, and as I watched, dark and brooding clouds surrounded the sun as it rose out of the ocean. I imagined they were angry now that Ames would no longer appear on that beach. But maybe she was still there. I finished my coffee and, already dressed in my running clothes, quietly went out the back door for one last run along the sand to bid farewell to Ames. As I ran toward the beach, the clouds lifted and the sun sent jewels sparkling across the ocean. Ames, I decided, was telling me that she was fine and not to worry. The tears clouding my eyes made it difficult to run.

When I returned to the house, it was coming alive with voices as everyone moved about the kitchen, grabbing a quick breakfast. We all said sad good-byes and headed back to our respective homes. Christmas was only a few weeks away, a good thing in my mind. The holiday season would keep us busy looking ahead to a less difficult time.

Or so I thought.

4

Christmas, Lee Style

When we returned to Baltimore and began preparations for Christmas, I again noticed nothing unusual about Lee. It was a busy time for him at the office. There were Christmas lunches with clients and office parties and year-end business dealings to tie up. He would return home in the evenings exhausted, but it seemed understandable, given the season.

We did manage to follow our usual routine of rising early to enjoy a cup of coffee together before I went for my run. I had no race ahead on the calendar, so I ran less intensely but still every day. As for Lee, his leg continued to bother him from the lump on his hamstring. Like any athlete with an injury, this made him irritable, especially because he still craved his daily exercise. So he rode the stationary bike in the basement or went to the pool for a swim. He would get a small burst of energy after his workout, but that seemed to quickly disappear into the commotion of the day. And, he was still coughing.

I became preoccupied with Christmas, my favorite holiday of the year. I loved stuffing the stockings that adorned our mantelpiece so that they overflowed with all sorts of goodies, necessities and the occasional embarrassing or humorous item. It was one of the few times of the year that we used our living room, making it that much more of a treasured time. The image of tiny lights sparkling on the tree in a room filled with laughter and gifts would resurrect happy childhood memories, even though my parents lived in two places.

My fantasy each year included being buttoned up in our house, shielded from the cold outdoors and, I hoped, snow, with the smell of wood burning in the fireplace. The magic of Christmas would lift everyone's spirits. I loved to spoil all three of my boys with special gifts and surprises and delicious meals.

The days leading up to this Christmas felt especially unsettling because my thoughts often wandered to Ames, plus I'd fallen behind in my Christmas preparations. I still hadn't bought a tree, and the boys were due to arrive in days. I wanted the tree up and dazzling when they got home, but something felt empty about decorating it alone after so many years of hanging ornaments as a family. Lee, though, was too busy at work after being away, and Tim wouldn't arrive from New York until Christmas Eve. Cryder—as was typical of him—had his last exam on the last possible day in the very last period. He then had to drive the five hours back from Chapel Hill. But at least he would be home for the full week before Christmas.

As luck would have it, a huge snowstorm was forecast to start in North Carolina around noon on the Friday Cryder would be driving home, and it was expected to travel north, just like him. So, already tired from studying for exams, he now faced the prospect of driving through a blizzard—a mother's nightmare. But I placed my faith in the fact that he had a big car and was a safe driver.

The storm hit as predicted, and Cryder got into his car at 5 p.m. and crawled his way up Interstate 95. It was a horrendous drive, but he knew that if he stopped, the roads would only get worse and he would be stuck in some hotel for the weekend. He ended up driving through the night while I worried and paced the house. He finally arrived at 5 a.m., snowplowing his way down the driveway with the fender of his car. I watched with my face pressed against the window, waiting to hug him as soon as he opened the front door.

When the snow finally stopped, we were buried, so we spent much of the weekend digging ourselves out. Although I liked the exercise, I noticed that I was doing most of the shoveling as Lee claimed exhaustion. It surprised me that he wasn't helping more. Still, it didn't matter. I was happy to have Cryder home and Christmas around the corner. And a white Christmas, too. Because of the snow, though, I fell even more behind schedule with my holiday preparations and final gift shopping, so my anxiety level increased. I had to get it all done. And Lee dragged; he simply wasn't his usual upbeat self. I decided that wrapping things up at the office in preparation for our post-Christmas trip had tuckered him out.

Christmas Eve arrived the next Thursday, and Tim was headed home on the train. We had a big party to attend that evening, the highlight of the weekend. It had become a tradition for many of our friends to gather that night, and I always enjoyed seeing all the boys' friends, adults now, and others we'd rarely see. When the boys were young, we raced home afterward, sent them to bed and then set about playing Santa, hanging stockings and laying out all the presents. But now that the boys were older, we stayed later at the party and got home around ten. Lee asked if we could just get up early in the morning to fill the stockings and arrange the gifts while the boys slept in. "I'm beat," he said. Agreed. I was tired, too.

That year, for the first time, we wouldn't be spending Christmas dinner with my mother, something I knew I'd miss. The many children and grandchildren always filled her house with the wonderful sounds, spirit, and chaos of the holidays. For the first few years that we lived next door to Mom and Jack, we spent Christmas morning with them, and then raced to New York City to have lunch with my father. It was hectic, but I loved the double Christmas. To me, Christmas has always been a time to celebrate love and family, and I had the opportunity to spend part of the day with both parents. After a few years, however, when the boys were still quite young and my dad now married to his third wife, things changed. Sadly, they stopped welcoming us when Tim was about four. Now I never see my father on Christmas or any other holiday and our communication usually only happens when I call him. It has left a hole in my heart, and makes me cherish my family even more.

When the four of us moved to Baltimore in 1994, we still spent our Christmas Eve and morning with the boys, but then we would climb in the car and drive the four hours or more it took to get to Long Island. There, many of my sisters, my brother, and some of the grand-children would be waiting for us. My husband was a very good sport about this, as were the boys, perhaps because the payoff was huge. Christmas dinner at Mom's was always a treat.

After so many years of making the trip, we decided to stay home the Christmas after Ames died. Lee just didn't seem to have the energy for the drive. I was crushed not to be with my family, but I certainly understood his desire to enjoy the long holiday weekend, just the four of us, without a long holiday car trip. And we had Tim home only until Sunday. I decided it was selfish of me to drag them away from our home every year so that I could keep alive the experience of Christmas with Mom. Besides, Lee and I had planned to return to Delray the Thursday after Christmas. While Lee flew back and forth to Baltimore for work, I'd be staying for the month of January to enjoy the warmth and our friends there, and to run more easily. After all, it was running that kept me sane—the constant in my life that gave me the strength to face life's obstacles.

In hindsight, I can see that I became passionate about running after my first full marathon in New York in 1985. I learned as I went and began watching other runners and studying their form. I listened to them explain their training routines, picked up racing tips, and tested their advice. And I searched through running magazines and periodi-cals I'd never noticed before. I became like a sponge, absorbing all the information I could get. I also sought out all kinds of races, from 5k's to marathons. There were local races within a forty-five-minute drive from our home almost every weekend. I began to dress the part too, discovering the lightweight running shoes and the less abrasive run-ning shorts and tops, allowing greater freedom of movement. And I began to place in those races, which inspired me for the next one. I had hardly known the world of running existed, and now I had discovered a hidden talent in that world. And a drive. The more I raced, the more I wanted to race.

Soon, I found myself consistently winning my age group. And then I began winning races overall. I became a target for the other local runners, who set their pace against mine and strove to beat me to the finish. The 5k's and 10k's were do-able on most weekends, but I knew I could only run a marathon once a year because of the time it took to train and the toll it would take on a runner's body. But the shorter races could be run throughout the year.

Much of my training was trial and error, and with a lot of error. I'd sometimes run very far on tired legs and find myself too far from home without the energy to return. In a race, the mistakes could be costly. If I went out too fast, for instance, I'd pay dearly with a death march to the finish. When I ran badly, I would beat myself up with criticism. But I learned much about myself from those experiences on the roads. I found I could increase my endurance by increasing my longer runs by a few miles each week. I found I could talk myself through the exhaustion, using my mind to help me overpower the fatigue, a message I was beginning to think I needed to instill in Lee. Mind over matter, I wanted to tell him.

I also discovered that my inner drive to compete was stronger than I'd ever thought. My desire to run, to race, to win had been waiting to be tapped. And I ran in all sorts of weather, from heat waves to snowstorms. There were days when I didn't think I could head out the door and days I didn't think I would make it home. But I pushed myself over and over again. And I always felt better about myself after I had run. *More messages I ought to convey to Lee*, I now thought, because back then, in the early days of running, my euphoria had been contagious.

It hadn't taken long before Lee, busy as he was, began to run, too. We had always played tennis for our exercise, and doubles for our social life. But now that I focused on running, he decided he needed to run in order to see me. Truth be told, when Tim was about two or three, I'd begun to worry about too much drinking on weekends, recalling my stepfather's bad drinking days before he went to AA, and asked Lee to stop. He turned over a new leaf and became as disciplined as I was. I think he saw that running reflected a healthier lifestyle, mentally as well as physically. He saw how running had given me confidence and a new sense of self. Running, I often told him, made me feel as if I could tackle anything. So Lee caught the bug too, and with my mother willing to watch Tim for us, our weekends began to fill with races instead of tennis.

Locally, I was getting a name for myself, and the recognition was a thrill. I won most of the races close to home; in Oyster Bay, Glen Cove, Jericho, Plainview and other places nearby. As I climbed the competitive ladder, Lee and I began to venture a little farther from home to race. The races were early-morning events on Saturdays or Sundays, so we got up before the sun rose and drove into Manhattan or to Connecticut or New Jersey in search of bigger challenges. Our weekend racing truly became a family affair when my mother decided that she and Tim wanted to watch us run. She took care of Tim while Lee and I ran our race, and then they would appear at the finish line to cheer us on.

We became part of a new "family," too, the running community itself, though at first it wasn't easy breaking into this new world. First of all, I became a threat to the women who used to win all the races. They didn't like being dethroned by this newcomer, nor did men like being passed by a woman. Lee, on the other hand, didn't care if I ran faster; he was all about meeting the challenges and loving the high after giving a race your all—the addiction factor. Second, they shunned me and tested me, throwing surges in on races (going at a faster pace for a short time to pull away from whoever is running with you) and cutting me off at water stops. Third, they ignored me. None of it scared me away. I worked to earn their respect and eventually, they acknowledged my presence and accepted both Lee and me.

Once that happened, we discovered a strong camaraderie among the runners, and many became our friends, transforming our weekend social life. Yes, we were competitive with each other, but we were also each other's greatest supporters. We encouraged each other on days we had bad races and congratulated each other on the good days. I found myself looking forward to seeing the women who were my fiercest competitors at the races. We had a great deal of respect for each other, and our friendships grew. There was, however, also a downside to this.

As those relationships blossomed, I sadly discovered that some, and I mean some, of my "old" friends came to resent my fame and my body, which had transformed into a sleek running machine. They hated when their husbands circled me at social events, asking about my running and how I trained, how I fit so much into my day of motherhood. The jealousies were hurtful, and eventually the fact that these women excluded Lee and me at weekend dinner parties upset me. But truly, when I look back, we were skipped over because they assumed we had no interest in dinner parties when we had races every weekend. That was our doing; one of the sacrifices we chose when racing became a priority.

I also felt guilty about taking Lee away from that life, though on occasion he experienced some jealousy of his own as he watched men surround me. A few times I found out exactly how he felt about these men long after the party. First, I'd sense his disdain, and then after I asked a few times what was bothering him, his Italian temper would flare a little. I assured him I only had eyes for him and jokingly asked who would put up with me anyway! But for the most part, Lee and I had gotten so caught up in the races that we hardly missed late nights and glasses of wine.

Occasionally, I entered a "big race," like the Women's 10k in Central Park, to test my ability against "the big girls." When I went to the starting line with all the famous runners, I watched them warm up with some easy jogging and a few sprints. I admired their physiques, and I was in awe of the way these runners seemed to soar effortlessly down the road, springing from step to step like gazelles. I watched and learned.

But my life as a runner was still centered on my family and being a wife and mother. The balance was important to me, and I wasn't willing to sacrifice my family time to focus solely on running. In fact, when Tim was three and attending a preschool two days a week, I switched careers and went to work with my mother. We bought an old house to renovate and sell. We had always done a good deal of handi-work and were both good at the cosmetic fixes around the house. We hired some contractors to work alongside us while we educated our-selves in the home renovation business. More learning by doing and observing.

The arrangement worked well in several ways. When Tim wasn't at school, I brought him to the house with his Fisher-Price tool set in his portable crib, and he "helped" us work. Then, while he took his three-hour afternoon nap, we worked some more. And during lunch, Mom gave me a free babysitting hour, picnicking with Tim while I went for my daily run. It all seemed to be working perfectly until, sur-prise, a new baby was on the way. The pregnancy thrilled Lee and me. I loved being a mom, which was really my biggest joy beyond any run-ning or racing. But it also meant that our competitive running would take a few months' break. I should add that Lee backed off his running a little in sympathy for me, so I wouldn't miss our old routine as much. He didn't compete again until I was back in shape and we could both enter races. Such a supportive husband! We did play plenty of tennis though. After all, we both had to get our exercise fix somehow.

5

Ill Health Rings In the New Year

Lee and I, in love with outdoor activity and warm weather, especially during the dreary East Coast winters, bought our condo near the ocean in Delray Beach in 2005. Initially, we only spent a few weeks there and rented the condo out so we could afford the cost. It was a long-term investment that we hoped to eventually spend more time in after retirement. But when Cryder left for college we began dedicating January as our time there, and whenever Lee joined me, we were "on the go" from dawn until dusk.

We typically started each day with my morning run and his bike ride, then hit the beach at lunchtime, and sometime later took a brisk forty-five-minute walk along the shore. Afterward, back at our apartment, I could usually persuade Lee to take another forty-five-minute bike ride on our cruisers, and then finish up with a little golf on the Par 3 course outside our door. Lee called it boot camp! For me, it was heaven. The only reason he looked forward to going back to Baltimore midweek was to get away from me, the drill sergeant.

In December of 2009, in light of Lee's lethargic behavior, I was especially eager to get him back into a healthy regimen. We arrived on the day before New Year's Eve without any definite plans to ring in 2010. Tim and his girlfriend, Gina, were coming down from New York to celebrate the new year and enjoy the weekend. They, of course, had their New Year's Eve all set—a black-tie party in Palm Beach, which made me quite jealous. I always love getting dressed up for a big black tie event.

Things seemed normal enough as Lee and I busily opened up the apartment and loaded the kitchen with food and drink. I was feeling guilty because Cryder had decided to stay at home in Baltimore to see his friends before heading back to UNC at the beginning of January to begin practicing for his last lacrosse season. We should have stayed with him, I thought more than once, as he rarely spent much time at home anymore. Though Lee made fun of me, I worried aloud about "our baby," all alone in our dark, cold house. Fortunately, we had Tim and Gina, and since they rarely visited I looked forward to our time together with them in Delray. Still, I wished I could have cloned myself, or Cryder!

Luckily for us, we ran into some friends from Baltimore who invited us to join their guests for New Year's Eve. Thank goodness—a party! I'm not a big fan of New Year's Eve, but I couldn't see us sitting alone in our apartment while everyone else was celebrating.

Tim and Gina flew into Fort Lauderdale, about forty miles south of Delray, and I had offered to pick them up and drive them directly to their party in Palm Beach, about twenty miles north of Delray. Lee grumbled about my offer because it meant we'd be in the car for a good two hours before heading to our party. To placate him, I said I'd drive and he could take a "roadie" and rest, something he usually agreed to. We also packed a small cooler in the car with some ice and wine so we could have a cocktail en route. Not, admittedly, the most responsible thing to do, but it was New Year's Eve.

It surprised me when Lee declined the wine and insisted on driving. Even when we were only ten minutes from home, he said he would wait to have a drink until we got to our party. Once again, he didn't seem to be acting like himself. What was wrong? Was he mad at me? It seemed like the wrong time to ask so I tried to be upbeat and excited about heading to the party.

We had this very handy moped that we kept in Delray. Lee thought it would work best to ride the moped the few miles to the party in downtown Delray, where parking might be an issue, and then it would also make it easier to scoot around and see the fireworks later. The main street, Atlantic Avenue, was being closed for a New Year's festival and fireworks show, and the evening's plans included everyone leaving the party before midnight and strolling to town to enjoy the festivities.

We arrived at the party a bit late and met a number of new people. Lee, usually very friendly and outgoing, seemed subdued as I listened to him mixing with others. I still worried that I had done something to annoy him. Once again, I was trying to be patient with my stubborn Italian husband, waiting for the right moment for him to speak his mind, or vice versa.

At about 11:30, everyone started moving to walk to town. Lee and I said we would meet them after riding in on the moped. As soon as we said our thank-yous and headed out the door, though, Lee asked if we could just go home. "I'm really tired," he said. "Maybe we can see some of the fireworks from our place."

"OK," I said, but it surprised me that he was ducking out. I asked again, "Is everything all right?"

"Yeah, just tired," he said.

We were home in about ten minutes and quietly headed into our place. We went out on the porch, watched a few fireworks and then went to bed. Midnight was late for both of us, even on New Year's Eve.

The weekend continued with lots of activity and beach time. Lee still seemed to be in another world, while I tried extra hard to be bubbly and upbeat to make up for his obviously low-key behavior. Tim had always been sensitive to his father's moods, and the last thing I wanted was for him to feel uneasy. Lee and I have always loved our long walks on the beach. We'd search for shells while we chatted about all sorts of things. He was being particularly quiet on one walk that weekend, though, and I finally said, "What's wrong with you? You're being so grumpy and unlike yourself. What is going on?"

He turned to me and brusquely replied, "I don't feel well. I am tired and have this annoying cough I can't get rid of."

"Then why don't you go to the doctor?" I snapped back. "You've been complaining about this 'cough' for months, and, frankly, it doesn't really seem like a bad cough to me. But get it checked. You haven't been yourself for a while, and I'm constantly on edge, worrying if I've done something wrong."

I don't think he was expecting my strong response. He'd been moping around like a helpless child, and I was fed up. I told him that he was putting a damper on the weekend with Tim and Gina and that he needed to make more of an effort. Lee's only real health issue, ever, was when both of his hips had been replaced in the same operation at the end of 2006, and I'd nursed him and kept him in good spirits during that ordeal. Now he apologized for having been bad-tempered and moody, but he also expressed frustration over his lack of energy and admitted he felt sorry for himself. He said he had made an appointment with his doctor on the Tuesday afternoon when he flew back to Baltimore.

"Good," I said. "It's about time."

We had one more night with Tim and Gina, and Lee made a huge effort to be outgoing. I knew he felt bad, and so did I for telling him off. But he knew that I could be like a lioness protecting her cubs when it came to me and my boys. I am not sure that Tim or Gina really noticed his lack of spunk, so I was probably overreacting—a weakness of mine, but I always want to make sure everyone's happy, a leftover from childhood and also fairly typical of middle children.

On the Monday after New Year's weekend, we dropped Tim and Gina at the airport, and then Lee and I had the day to ourselves. We went for our usual walk on the beach, and he tried hard to keep up. Then we rode our bikes and after that played a quick nine holes of golf. We had a quiet dinner at home. He told me he was anxious to get to the doctor to learn why he felt so exhausted all the time.

"Maybe you have mono or maybe you're low in iron," I suggested.

Lee said the doctor was going to do some blood work, adding, "I'm going to ask him to check this lump on my leg again because it's still aching all the time."

"Please do," I said, "because we need to get you back into shape. You have to be able to keep up with me at 'boot camp'!"

On Tuesday morning, I took Lee to the airport. I would enjoy the time by myself in Delray—running to my heart's content, sitting and reading on the beach, having a simple soup-and-salad dinner. Still, I felt lonely when he left and most certainly missed my best friend's company.

Later that afternoon, Lee called to say his appointment went well. The doctor took some blood samples and gave him a full physical. The doctor said he was pretty sure that the ache in his leg was a hamstring tear that would heal in time. A hamstring tear? "When did you tear your hamstring?" He thought it must have happened when he was dancing at the wedding in November. "Wow, I don't remember you dancing that crazy, or saying anything about it the night of the wedding. It wasn't until the morning that you said your leg was sore." Now I felt guilty because I'd given him a hard time about his "sore leg," but I remained skeptical about the doctor's diagnosis because a hamstring tear doesn't usually appear as a lump. Also, if it tears, you definitely feel that, and Lee didn't remember any sudden pain. So be it, I eventually decided, he's the doctor.

Lee was only in Baltimore for the one night, flying back down on Wednesday evening because Cryder and his girlfriend were visiting for a few days before they headed back to UNC for the spring semester. This was their only chance to come down because lacrosse started in less than a week for both of them—she played on the women's team at UNC too—and there would be no more vacation time for them after that.

During Cryder's visit, I mentioned to him that Lee had a persistent and annoying cough and felt rundown. We had our private chuckle about how helpless Lee could be when feeling sick, but I also told

Cryder that the doctor had ran some blood tests and we were waiting to hear. I was obviously concerned, but I still thought his malaise must be due to something simple, like an iron deficiency. After all, we were a healthy family, and we made a point of staying that way.

6

Two Wins and a Scare

From the time Lee and I met we always included sports in our lives. In college we ran together while I was getting in shape for lacrosse season. After we married in 1980, we began playing a lot of tennis. Everyone in my family was an avid tennis player. Luckily, Lee had great hand-eye coordination and caught on quickly, since my sisters loved to test any man who dared to step on the court, firing shots to see how fast he could react. I know—not very nice—but it was amusing! We also skied whenever we could. Lee was a beautiful skier and had been the captain of his high school ski team. And then there was our running and his golf.

Our sports activities, especially my running, became more challenging after we had Cryder, our second son. On a very hot day in June 1987, about a week before Cryder was born, Lee and I played in our last tennis tournament. I felt wobbly after the game and a little light-headed. Lee noticed and threw up his hands. "Enough!" he insisted, and for once I agreed. No wonder Cryder arrived four days early—he wanted out of my nonstop body! Tim had been hoping for a little brother, and much to Tim's content, we were blessed with a healthy baby boy. The day after Cryder's birth, Lee came to the hospital with a box of new running shoes for me—the best present ever. He knew that I couldn't wait to get back into my running routine.

With two children to care for, fitting in the running meant I had to be extremely organized, and my times to train needed to be quality runs, not just what runners call "junk miles," or runs to increase mileage. I didn't have time for that. I was very focused on the running I needed to fit in, but I was also very focused on being a mom. As much as I prided myself on being a good runner, being a good mom and wife were the most important things to me. Because of my parents' divorce, I had made a vow that my family always came first; that was priority number one.

I managed my time well, with my mother still helping when she could. Life became even better when we moved into a house right next door to my parents in Mill Neck in July of 1988, just after Cryder's first birthday and before Tim's fifth. Mom turned into a second mother to our boys, who couldn't wait to run up the path to their grandparents' house. That, of course, worked well for me, giving me more free time. Making cookies at grandma's could take several hours at least!

Before long, I was back in shape and my running times began falling. My success grew, and again I found myself seeking out more competitive events, testing myself against faster women. I continued to learn more about what my body was capable of doing; push through the pain, endure it and my body would amazingly become stronger. And nationally, I was climbing in the ranks of runners, with 5k times of around 17:30 minutes and 10k's of around 37 minutes, each within a minute or so of competitive national times.

Then one day, in 1988, one of my mother's younger brothers, Bobby, suggested something that would test my body in a new way. Bobby, an avid runner who lived near Boston, had been running the Boston Marathon for more than fifteen years. But now he had found a new challenge: a triathlon. He had plans to travel with a group that would be racing in September. He called and invited me to join them. What exactly, I asked, would this triathlon involve?

I had heard of an Ironman before, and I hoped he wasn't talking about that! He explained that not all triathlons involve Ironman distances, just as not all road races are marathons. The Bermuda race would be an Olympic distance course—a .9-mile swim, followed by a 26-mile bike ride, topped off with a 6.2-mile run. He piqued my curiosity. What kind of person would do that? Would I? Could I? Why not? I said yes.

As for Lee, he thought it sounded like fun, something that would challenge me. Since I loved running, why not expand that into a triathlon? I'd been a pretty good swimmer as a child and I enjoyed biking. I even had a bike in college, which I used daily to commute to classes and lacrosse practice. That is, until it got stolen and I couldn't afford a replacement. Lee had no interest in training with me at that point, though both of us looked forward to going to Bermuda, a place that held special memories for us. It was where Lee and I spent our college spring break in 1977 when he first confessed he had fallen in love with me, and of course I had fallen in love with him from almost the moment I met him!

However, adding two more sports to my already busy schedule meant even more juggling, and that did concern us. I had to be careful not to throw the kids at him the minute he walked through the door. Lee worked hard, so I had to pick my times carefully and make sure he hadn't had a bad day at the office. Boys, in particular, can be rambunctious and trying.

What also proved challenging was that I didn't own a bike, nor had I swum any laps in years. My uncle Bobby said he would lend me a ten-speed bike and a helmet. The swimming was my real problem. I had about three and a half months to prepare, just like for my first 10-mile Boston Marathon run with Kitty. I relearned how to swim laps and trained myself to ride a bike again. The first few times out on the bike were not as easy as I'd imagined; I hadn't used those muscles in a long time. I thought the strength I gained from running would easily transition into cycling, but I soon realized that the different motion, that of pulling and pushing the pedals, was tiring my legs quickly. The same thing happened when I swam laps, only worse. I may have thought I was in such great shape, but it was difficult trying to exercise and hold my breath at the same time. And swimming was more upper body work, muscles I certainly had not called upon for years. This new sport was going to take some work!

I spent most of the time training by myself. Many of the runners I met trained with other runners, but usually in the evenings when I had my children to take care of and husband to cook for. As when I'd learned running techniques, I now asked others about training for triathlons, and Bobby gave me a few tips. The Internet still belonged to the future, though I did read running magazines and tried to adapt what I learned to biking and swimming. Mainly, though, my teacher was trial and error.

At the end of August, I ran into a friend who told me about a sprint triathlon in early September in Bayville, a few weeks before the Bermuda event. It was right down the road from our house and would be a perfect test to see what I'd gotten myself into. The distance included a half-mile swim, a 15-mile bike ride, and then a 5k run. I'd been training for a longer race, so this would be a good trial run.

That morning, I arrived at this small-town race with my mom, Lee, and our two sons. Metal racks were lined up in the parking lot for the athletes to stow their bikes. I noticed the athletes had laid towels on the ground next to their bikes, along with buckets of water, running shoes, helmets, glasses, and extra shorts. I didn't have any of this stuff. I wandered over to a couple in the midst of spreading out their things and explained that this was my first race—would they mind helping me? What's the plastic bucket of water for? To dip your sandy feet into after running up the beach from the swim and before putting on your shoes, they explained patiently. Though once they said it, the obviousness of it made me think I should have known. They also showed me how to roll my socks back to just the toe so my damp foot wouldn't get stuck when I tried to put each sock on. I thanked them for all their help and set my own things up. I only had my bike, helmet, and running shoes, which I placed on the paved spot next to my bike. I'd have to improvise the rest.

I checked in with the volunteers and they wrote my number on my legs and arms. Since you can't wear a paper number swimming, that's how they keep track of you coming out of the water. I stood at the edge of the beach, fearful yet anxious to get the race started. I had no idea what it would be like to run the fifty yards down the beach, dive into the water, and swim around the buoys marking the swim course along with so many other athletes.

The gun finally went off and I dashed down the sandy beach toward the water with the others, trying to keep my own space. Elbows were flying as we raced to the water, high stepping through the shallow part until we were far enough out to dive in. Then suddenly I was swimming with bodies all around me. It was terrifying. Each time I went to take a breath someone seemed to be pushing me, fighting for space, too. I tried to keep calm, telling myself to keep swimming—don't stop or you'll be drowned! I started to get into a rhythm, and then, before I knew it, the half-mile ended and I was thankfully running back up the beach. I knocked some sand off my feet with my socks, then put them on and was off on my bike.

The bike ride involved a very flat loop around town, and it seemed to go by quickly. I had no idea of my position in the race, I just kept riding. When I passed my family, I briefly caught their cheers as the wind rushed past my ears. Getting off my bike and starting to run was another story. I was not prepared for how shaky my legs were or how numb my feet felt as I tried to set my usual pace. It took a few minutes until the familiar sensation returned, of one foot and then the next comfortably hitting the pavement. As I approached a few young women in front of me, I felt a surge of adrenaline and quickened my pace. Then I began to pass other runners, and my excitement grew. I was gaining ground, steadily hunting down the women in front of me. With just about a half mile to go, I passed the only other women left in front of me. I could hear the spectators cheering for me: "First woman! Way to go! Finish is right around the corner!"

My family, waiting by the finish line, cheered wildly. They couldn't believe I had come in first—nor could I. I was thirty years old. I beamed! Of course, my husband had an inkling what this meant, and we shared a knowing smile—another new sport. But Lee was also proud of me for winning my first triathlon, and winning this race gave me a tremendous boost and newfound enthusiasm for the Bermuda Triathlon. I could hardly wait to hear the pop of the starting gun. Little did we know that Lee would soon catch the triathlon bug too!

～ ～ ～

Lee's doctor finally called on Friday, January 8, 2010. He said the blood test showed a low red-blood-cell count, indicating some kind of infection. He wanted Lee to come back in for more blood work when he returned to Baltimore. That, I hoped, would determine exactly what was wrong and get Lee quickly back to his old self. After the nonstop activity of the previous ten days we had a quiet weekend—playing golf, riding bikes, walking, and then turning in early each night.

On Monday morning, Lee flew home and went straight to his office. Tuesday morning he stopped by the lab to give more blood, and Thursday night he arrived back in Delray to help me entertain. My stepsister Wendy—best friend, sweet, kind, and fun-loving—and her husband, Jeff, were coming down from their home in Hilton Head for the weekend to play in a golf tournament with us. (This tournament was on a par three eighteen-hole course, so not that demanding, and we did very little walking.) Lee and I adored both Wendy and Jeff, so I thought their visit would be a good distraction for both of us. Results from the latest blood work, we hoped, would come soon. Waiting was not my strong suit!

We shared many laughs with Wendy and Jeff that weekend as we caught each other up on our lives, with the exception of Lee's health issues. As a very private guy, he preferred not to bring it up. He did his best to be cheerful, but I could tell he was struggling. When we went out late on Saturday night, he once again grew quiet and seemed annoyed. He insisted he felt exhausted and couldn't shake the cobwebs. All weekend, I kept quietly asking, "Any calls from the doctor?" Nothing.

In the meantime, I had been discussing Lee's situation with Barbara Crocker, my new best friend in Florida and a fellow runner. She and I had often crossed paths as we ran the roads of Delray for the past five or so years. She is a wisp of a woman, probably about five foot two and no more than ninety pounds, while I'm a six-foot-tall giant with strawberry-blonde hair. After a while, we recognized each other as we passed and we would smile and wave, but I only finally met her because of Tim.

The year before, while in Delray, Tim had gone to visit his friend Sara, and the topic of running came up as he chatted with Sara's mother, Barbara. Tim told her, "You've probably seen my mom. Everyone always sees her running—she runs everywhere." When Tim described me, Barbara said she passed me every morning, knew exactly who he meant, and wanted to meet me. A day or two later, I was running down the road and saw, way ahead, a woman running toward me, madly waving and screaming, "I'm Barbara!" Tiny woman, enormous personality. We stopped, chatted, and became fast friends.

Barbara had been in Delray for more than twenty-five years and actually lived right around the corner from us. She was also an emailing and texting machine, and we found ourselves communicating constantly, although there was no way I could keep up with her machinegun speed on the keypad or the volume of her emails. Whenever I arrived in Delray, I would send Barbara an "I'm here" email, and we'd look for each other on our familiar running route. Runners often share an instant connection, and it happened like that for us. With Barbara, I immediately shared life secrets, concerns, and stories, and so from the start I sent her an email about Lee's health issues:

Lee is still coughing and feeling tired. The tests came back inconclusive. His white blood cells are still elevated, and the doc is thinking it's some kind of infection. He's on antibiotics and has to go back to see him as soon as he gets home. Weird.

She wrote back: "Sure antibiotics will help—that and being with you so you can take care of him."

Her support was exactly what I needed as Lee and I waited for the results. I needed reassurance from someone.

Wendy and Jeff left Sunday morning amid promises to stay in better touch, and as soon as they were gone, Lee headed for our apartment, saying he was exhausted and wanted to take a nap. He had already slept in late, so I was hoping we could go for a long walk on the beach. I settled for a bike ride by myself.

When I came back, Lee was happily sitting on the sofa getting ready to watch some football. It was an overcast day, a good day for watching a game, which I agreed to do with him if we could play a game of twilight golf later. We loved our twilight golf. All we needed to do to play was step out of our first floor apartment. And we usually had the small course to ourselves, at least in a way. We always thought we were alone, until we'd hear the sliding doors of our condo neighbors— whoosh, whoosh—and then a shout of "good shot" or "tough putt!"

A huge breakthrough occurred for me in the Bermuda Triathlon. Though racing in the Bayville Triathlon had boosted my confidence, I admit that I felt a bit scared and daunted by the approaching Bermuda event. The fact that we needed to fly to the pretty island, located several hundred miles off the East Coast, complicated the mere act of traveling. Before the trip, I had to take the bike apart and pack it up in an old carton that a bike shop down the road had given me. On the appointed day, all my gear was checked in and loaded onto the plane for the three-hour flight across the Atlantic. At the other end of our trip, my uncle, familiar with this process, had promised to help me reassemble the bike. That is, if the bike didn't get lost on the way to Bermuda. We were warned of that possibility.

We had a free family place to stay in Bermuda, and a few family members would be staying there too. My mother insisted she join us as our loyal supporter. Several of my cousins had signed up for the race, too, and she said she wanted to cheer them on, as well. Lee, of course, accompanied me as the leader of my cheering squad, but Tim and Cryder stayed behind, mostly due to considerations of cost. This was one of the few times they'd stay home as I hated to leave my children and missed them the entire trip. It did, however, make for fewer distractions and allowed me to conserve energy and stay focused on my mission—I had to make it to the finish line of this race.

Fortunately, my bike arrived without a hitch, and Uncle Bobby helped me to assemble it. On race day, however, I was a bundle of nerves. It turned out that this was a big race in the triathlon world, and all the stars were there. This triathlon also included separate professional and amateur divisions, the difference being that the pros competed for cash winnings and world ranking, whereas the amateurs competed amongst themselves for overall and group placement. Considering how many more athletes would race in Bermuda than in Bayville, I immediately began to worry about the swim; all those flailing arms and legs, the pushing and shoving, and nearly a mile in choppy waters, no less. It would be rough.

When I went to find my spot on the bike rack and, this time, position my towel on the ground next to my bike, I looked around to see how others had set things up. These athletes were a different breed from the people I had raced against back on Long Island. Their bikes were sleek, deluxe models with special wheels and handlebars—clearly very fast. My clunky bike couldn't compare. Even their helmets looked fancier! Their helmets fit like gloves, shiny and oblong shaped, while mine looked like a giant white mushroom atop my head. I felt out of place in this big pond. The athletes—both the pros and the amateurs—tinkered with their bikes and examined and reexamined their gear. And everything they had they lined up just right. I tried to do the same, peeking at them now and then to be sure I at least looked like I knew what I was doing.

While I waited on the beautiful pink sand for my turn to dash into the water, I felt ready to throw up. Nerves, nerves, nerves! I just wanted the race to start. *Breathe deep, try to make your body relax*, I reminded myself, but thinking about the swim petrified me. And I was right—it proved awful. I swallowed a ton of salt water, and my goggles leaked just enough to allow the salty water to sting my eyes. I hit gobs of seaweed, getting it caught around my arms, but I swam the 9-mile 0.9 course, ran back onto the beach, brushed some of the sand off my feet, and charged toward my bike.

The 26-mile bike course proved very difficult, but I managed to navigate the hilly, winding roads before trudging my way through the incredibly hot and humid 6.2-mile run. Climbing up the last, endlessly long hill toward the finish line at the Southampton Princess resort, I was pouring sweat and my lungs burned as I gasped for air in the densely humid air. My legs felt ready to buckle and with each foot strike my quads burned. But the cheers of the crowd suddenly began drawing me faster and faster.

Because the race had been set off in waves instead of a mass start, no one knew their final position until it was announced. As for me, I had no idea what place I finished, nor did I really care—I was just happy to have crossed the finish line. I also failed to realize they had an awards ceremony a few hours after the race. Nor had it occurred to me that I might even win something!

Not until late afternoon, when one of my cousins returned with the results, did I discover how I'd done. My name appeared at the top of a list: I had won the women's amateur division! As in WON! I was truly shocked and elated. More than elated, though also disappointed when I learned that I'd missed the big awards ceremony where the winners were called on stage to collect their trophies.

Of course, my mother and Lee were thrilled for me. In fact, Lee took half the credit as my number one cheerleader! But some of the other family members, who'd also competed, seemed a little less than happy for me. Congratulations occurred through gritted teeth, but I was now learning how to deal with jealousies and did my best to be cordial.

A funny thing happened the following morning. We had to call one of the race directors to coordinate picking up my trophy. At about

9 a.m., Lee called the man, who sounded quite groggy. It seemed he'd had a wonderful time celebrating the night before, another event we hadn't known about and also had missed. In any case, off we drove on a moped, one of the preferred methods of getting around the island. Once we found the home of this man, he handed us a huge box containing a watermelon-sized Waterford Crystal Bowl with Bermuda International Triathlon and 1st Place—Amateur Female engraved on it. Up to that point most of my awards had been plastic gold statues of runners. Now we were faced with the additional problem of transporting this huge box on the back of a moped. Although it almost caused us to topple a few times, I hung onto it for dear life, and to this day that beautiful sparkling bowl sits on a glass shelf in our dining room china cabinet.

I really didn't know what this win meant for my future running career. In particular, I did not yet see my running as a "career"; especially not triathlons, not with two young children. How could I consistently find time to train for three sports when I hardly had the time to train for one? Moreover, we were unaware that triathlons took place all over the country and the world. At that point, as far as I was concerned, this Bermuda Triathlon was a one-time race and I would return to running.

7

More Tests to Endure

January 2010

No sooner had Wendy and Jeff left Delray than my sisters Edie and Nini came to visit for two nights. Lee had returned to Baltimore, where he had more blood work lined up after the previous tests had come back with no diagnosis, so us girls had three days to ourselves, a welcome distraction for me because I was increasingly concerned about Lee.

But the time with my sisters was perfect, a healing time. Nini still struggled with the loss of her twin, and Edie, being the nurturing older sister, was very sensitive to her. Edie, though, was also hurting as she had been the one who'd taken care of Ames through her hard times, and now, still living in the same town as Ames had, she didn't get through a day without feeling her loss. But we spent our few days together as siblings once again, giggling, teasing each other, and reminiscing.

Still, my sisters could sense something was troubling me, so I finally filled them in on Lee's puzzling fatigue and cough. Empathetic to my concern, they speculated on the diagnosis. Nini had had Lyme disease twice and thought that's what it must be, and the lab, in fact, was testing for Lyme disease that week. Edie and Nini both assured me that Lee would be fine—he was, after all, a tough guy who had survived all of us Cushing girls during his college years and beyond.

All too soon, Edie and Nini left, and Lee was arriving back in town—followed by more houseguests, a common occurrence when you have a place in Florida! I raced around cleaning up again. Lee and I had a couple of days to ourselves until our best friends from our early married days, John and Dianne Smith, came to visit from Long Island. They'd be there from Saturday to Monday. We were godparents to each other's children and shared much history together. We had managed to stay close friends over the years despite our living so far away.

During their visit, we had beach time, golf, and relaxed dinners, from burgers and fries at the Office to fresh fish at City Oyster. I ached from laughing, and Lee rallied for their visit. By now, in fact, he'd tired of talking about his blood tests and fatigue. Lee was usually on his game with John, loving to needle him, which generally improved his mood. Still, I watched him more carefully, determined to figure out his mysterious fatigue. On Monday, after John and Dianne left, the afternoon was free. But again, Lee ducked out of our afternoon bike ride and opted for a nap. When I came back, he asked if I wanted to go for a little walk.

"Of course I do!" I exclaimed.

We headed to the end of the road by the Intracoastal Waterway for the sunset, which Lee and I loved to watch. That day a particularly beautiful display of orange and pink colors spread across the horizon. He was leaving again in the morning for Baltimore, and I had the next three days to clean the apartment, this time for our February and March renters. As Lee and I enjoyed the sunset, we held hands and talked about what a great place we had in Delray and how much we always hated to leave it. Somehow, though, I sensed that Lee wanted to say something else. To this day I can still picture us standing at the water's edge as Lee turned to me and said, "My doctor wants me to check into the hospital when I get back to Baltimore."

"Are you serious? Why didn't you say something earlier?" My heart was suddenly racing.

Lee didn't answer my questions. He simply said, "The doctor wants me to have a bone marrow test."

I felt myself sway and was suddenly yanked away from the beauty of the sunset to fear tingling through my bloodstream.

"I'm going home with you," I said immediately.

"No," Lee said emphatically. "Don't be ridiculous. You have to get the apartment ready. The bone marrow test won't be until Wednesday and the results probably won't come back until you're home anyway. They're only trying to rule things out. They want me to check in because that way all the tests can be done in one place, and they get done more quickly." Apparently, his red blood cell count had continued to drop and they planned to run several blood tests checking for everything from various infectious blood diseases to Hodgkin's lymphoma.

I was shocked and didn't know what to say. I had so much to do to get our place ready, but I didn't want him sitting in a hospital room without me to keep him company. He insisted, though, saying he'd probably only be in the hospital for twenty-four hours, and I would be home in just a few days anyway. He would be fine, and I should stop worrying.

When I dropped Lee off at the airport early Tuesday morning, I wanted to leave the car and go with him. But, again, he insisted he'd be fine. He promised he would be. We'd meet at the airport in Baltimore on Friday afternoon, and then we would fly together to Chapel Hill for Cryder's first lacrosse scrimmage of the season at seven o'clock that night.

Barbara Crocker had returned to Georgetown where she also had an apartment, so I had lost my running companion during all this, but she provided support through our constant emailing. And when I told her Lee had checked in at the Greater Baltimore Medical Center, she offered to go there immediately to be my eyes and ears and to bring Lee some of her delicious homemade chicken soup. Though kind of her to offer, I knew Lee wanted his privacy.

In the middle of all this, I decided the boys needed to know what was happening. Lee and I had previously decided it wasn't necessary to tell them about all the testing until we had some answers. Lee didn't want to worry them—but a bone marrow test? The thought frightened me, so I decided that the time had come to tell them about the situation. Mid-afternoon that Tuesday, I emailed them:

January 26, 2010

Hey, guys. Wanted to update you on Dad's situation. He was admitted into GBMC today so they can do some more testing. He had twelve vials of blood taken last week to test for everything from hepatitis, lymes, etc. Everything came back negative. His red blood cell count is still going down, so they are now going to do some bone marrow testing.

I know, that's scary, but he says they have to start trying to rule things out like Hodgkin's, etc. I just wanted to let you know what was going on. I'm sure he's a bit nervous too. He told me last night he was seeing some specialists, including an oncologist, which flipped me out and I told him I wanted to go back with him. He insisted it is all precautionary and they are just trying to figure things out.

I sent some flowers to his room from all of us to cheer him up. He'll probably get mad at me for telling you guys all this, but I thought it was best to keep you updated. Don't worry, he's a tough old ginny!! Love you guys.

Xox

I was also trying to keep Edie and Nini up-to-date as I needed and wanted my sisters' support and reassurance. (My mother and Jack were out of the country for a few weeks, so I was relying on my sisters more than usual.) Edie wrote a lovely thank you note for her visit, and I responded with our news. As always, Edie was full of positive thoughts, and it made me feel better to know she was there.

Still, I felt so helpless in Delray and was mad at myself that Lee had persuaded me to stay put. I really should have been there with him, since he had always been there for me. So throughout those few days, to overcome my fears about what might be going on with Lee,

I ran as much as possible. That's when I could think more clearly, make a plan, and reason that he was fine. Besides, my mind grows peaceful when I run—my feet pounding the pavement, my breath entering and exiting, just me and my thoughts. Everything will be okay.

8

Triathlons Are Contagious

It had been my fate as a runner to become an endurance machine—somewhat indestructible, definitely determined—and I was about to find out why.

During the winter following the Bermuda Triathlon in 1988, which I'd won, Lee and I went up to New Hampshire for a family ski trip. As a group of us sat around the table after dinner enjoying some wine, I noticed some intense conversation between Lee and my uncle Bobby. Bobby had come up with another enticing idea: how about we all go to Saint Croix in May and compete in the America's Paradise Triathlon?

I looked at Lee, hoping he'd say yes, while in fact he was hoping I would. After discussing it later and perhaps encouraged by the wine and the lure of the Caribbean island, we jumped on board that night. But this race would be an even a bigger challenge than the Bermuda Triathlon, for it was double the distance. In other words, it was a half Ironman, consisting of a 1.2-mile swim, a 56-mile bike ride, and a 13.1-mile run—each as fast as you can go. This time, Lee decided he'd participate in the race, not just cheerlead. What were we getting into now? Bobby assured us that five months was plenty of time to train.

Just as we'd been running in races together before, the preparation for this triathlon once again became a family affair. Lee had given me a ten-speed bike for Christmas and had bought himself one too, so at least this time I had my own bike. We did not have a coach—no money in the budget for that—but we trained by simply doubling the distances that I'd used when I trained for Bermuda, figuring that since I had done well such a strategy would work. In fact, our training was far below what it should have been. We biked maybe three times a week, with our longest ride being around 35 miles, not nearly long enough; we swam two to three times per week, maybe as much as a mile at a time; and we ran five to six times a week, running being the easiest to fit into our schedules. We ran, biked, and swam until we thought we were ready for this big event.

This time my mom stayed home with the children, and Lee and I set out on our adventure to Saint Croix with our bikes and gear in tow. It was not an easy way to travel, and it seemed like an awful lot of stuff for our short three-day stay, but that was all the time we could afford.

When we arrived in Saint Croix at the beginning of May, we found the weather much hotter and far more humid than we had expected, hardly bearable for racing (though we'd checked the temperature we hadn't thought to check the humidity level), and now we had no extra time on the island to acclimate to the heat. Making the whole experience even more formidable, both the bike race and the run were on extremely hilly and winding roads, an unbelievably challenging course. We both were more than a little scared!

On the morning of the race, we took a small ferry out to the tiny island where the swim would start. This was a major professional race, so it had attracted many of the top professionals in the sport and would include more than six hundred participants. Looking around at all the fit bodies, Lee and I were totally intimidated. We felt outclassed. Next, we wandered around a corner to check if we could see where the bright orange buoys marked the swim course, and we did: they stretched out beyond our line of sight. I took a deep breath and stated the obvious to Lee: "That is a long, long way!" In this race, I decided I was no longer concerned about where I'd place—my only hope was to finish.

Once again, I had the pre-swim butterflies, envisioning all those bodies surrounding me in the water. My wave of racers, about seventy-five of us, was to leave before Lee's, so I gave him a hug and kiss, and we wished each other good luck. "Be careful out there," I said, and then I was off, knowing I had to follow my own advice, especially at the start.

You see, there is an enormous amount of initial jockeying for position and thrashing around for space in the water. Once the swimmers were spread out enough I no longer felt crowded. But a new problem emerged about halfway through the swim: the pressure around my eyes from the goggles was killing me. Not long afterward, the sensation became so excruciating that I had to stop and tread water and take the goggles off to relieve the pain. Obviously I had them on too tight, but how could I fix that now? No, I had to put them back on, endure the pain and keep swimming. I remember shifting my thoughts, distracting myself from the agony and looking down at the bottom of the deep blue ocean, thinking there must be some really giant fish down there. Maybe sharks? By terrifying myself I inadvertently did a good job of making myself swim faster and faster. Sharks would be a lot worse than those stupid goggles. Once I reached the shore I ripped those goggles off my head as fast as I could.

My adrenaline was pumping as I raced toward my bike for the next leg of the half Ironman. I was happy to be on dry land, but the hills and the heat were brutal. The race was subtitled "The Beauty and the Beast," and I now understood why, particularly when I had to dismount my bike and walk it, serpentine style as most other athletes did, up the unbelievably long steep hill. It was that difficult to climb.

With 40 miles behind me and 15 miles to go, the course rounded the island and we were biking dead into the wind. Suddenly, my bike seemed to be going nowhere. My mind screamed at my legs to pedal but I couldn't make the bike go any faster. The wind tore at me. *Keep pedaling*, I told myself; what else was there to do?

Somehow I made it to the end of the course, and I couldn't get rid of that bike fast enough! Now only the run remained. *One segment left. I can do this*, I thought to myself. Dismounting my bike was a shock to my legs as they felt wobbly and my feet felt numb. *Keep moving*, I told myself as my hobbling turned to running and I began to feel more in control. Soon, my body seemed to move with a spirit of its own, even though fatigue was exerting its own opposite pull.

The run had some out-and-back sections, allowing us to see other runners as well as the competition. I was making ground during the run, and my legs finally seemed to find themselves as I urged myself forward. On the way to the turnaround, I saw my younger cousin heading back toward town, and he was running strong. We shared a thumbs-up. When I made the turn, I looked for Lee amid the runners coming toward me on the other side of the road. I worried about him, though maybe he worried about me too. This was so much harder than I'd expected, and this was his first time. Whose idea had this been anyway!?

About ten of our friends and family had entered this race—all of whom had finished several triathlons before—and they too were struggling with Saint Croix's terrain. That worried me even more. Every time I spotted one of our gang coming toward me on the way back to town, I would scream, "Have you seen Lee?" But no one had.

I ran a little faster now. I could sense the end near, giving me another rush of adrenaline. My body was glistening with sweat, with beads of salty water streaming down my face. One last hill to climb and then I'd head down King Street to the finish line. Everyone, local islanders as well as all the athletes' supporters, cheered madly while steel drums played. I pushed myself toward the finish line, and, as soon as I crossed, my legs buckled. I let exhaustion take over. And then I glanced at the clock: it read six hours, two minutes.

In my age group, I had finished fifth, and while the time was average overall, it was competitive among the women, and for me particularly, considering it was my first half Ironman. I now knew that I hadn't been physically prepared enough for this grueling race, and yet at the same time I was elated that, somehow, my determination had pushed my body to finish. I was both exhausted and pumped knowing I'd succeeded.

Once my breathing regulated, I went directly to the transition area where all the bikes were racked. Luckily, I passed tables stacked with cups of water, which I desperately drank or dumped over my head to cool down. Knowing where Lee's bike had been positioned, I searched to see if it was there, and it was, which meant he had made it back from the ride. Strewn about the bike were his helmet, goggles, and cap. Phew! This meant he was out on the run course.

I turned to watch the runners coming in, straining to find Lee, trying to guess where he might be. It seemed a very long time before I spotted him, cresting the last hill at the top of King Street. He was still running, a bit more slowly than usual, but still running. And as he ran toward the finish line, he wore a big grin and lifted his hand up, high-fiving the spectators. I was so relieved to see him still smiling. It took him over seven hours, but he did it. He was ecstatic, and I was very proud: what an introduction to triathlons!

That summer after the Saint Croix triathlon, Lee and I began serious triathlon training, though still without a coach. We learned from other athletes and from current magazines on the sport that we needed to increase the distance of our practices in all three areas—swimming, biking, and running. We swam, biked, and ran longer distances in our practices than what we'd face in a race—a 10-mile run, for example, for an actual 10k segment of a race. We also ran, biked, and swam more frequently. Through strengthening and conditioning, we built up our stamina. With the children either in tow or on occasion with their grandmother, we traveled two to three times a month in Long Island, Connecticut, New Jersey, and even New Hampshire to race in triathlons of varying lengths.

It was a lot, but we thrived on both the healthy benefits of the training and the races themselves. An added benefit was that family members came to watch us, and our sons developed an appreciation for the rigors of competitive sports. They even worked at the water stops and on occasion accompanied us to the podium to collect trophies. Of course there were also times when they would rather have been elsewhere!

Triathlons encompass a season that stretches until mid-October, and by then we were both ready to take a break until it started up again in spring. I still ran a few races throughout the winter to keep in shape.

In 1991, my racing became increasingly serious. At that time, when Cryder was four and attending the same elementary school as Tim, I switched careers again. The housing market had crashed in New York and the business with my mom had struggled. I became a part-time coach working in the afternoons at the boys' school, where I coached the fifth- to ninth-grade girls in soccer, basketball, and lacrosse. It was rewarding to work with the girls, and the schedule allowed me to keep up with my morning training. Cryder's day was not as long as Tim's, so he often joined me on the field or in the gym to "help" me, as Tim had with our house renovation, or Mom would come by several afternoons a week to take him back to her house. A mom is a mom is a mom!

Competing in triathlons required a disciplined training schedule, which I created without the assistance of a coach, a luxury we still couldn't afford. I based mine on schedules I read about in triathlon magazines, modified to fit the other demands on my time—being a mom and working part-time. Essentially, I ran four to five days a week, usually between five and seven miles, with one longer day of twelve to thirteen miles. But that was only the running, the least time-consuming aspect. I biked the same number of days as I ran: ten- to fifteen-mile rides, with one of about twenty to thirty miles. The pool I used for my practices was located twenty-five minutes from home, making this the most difficult sport to deal with, but I tried to get a one-mile swim in at least three times a week.

Triathlons also proved expensive, what with all the required travel and equipment. But my disciplined training soon bore results. I rose in the competitive ranks, finding myself racing at regional, national, and even world championships. And when I placed among the top women, the prize money helped cover most expenses of the sport we loved.

As I became better known in multisport circles, I was also lucky enough to receive sponsorship offers from various companies. Saucony gave me running shoes, Aegis donated bikes, handlebars came from Vision Tech, racing wheels from Hed Wheels, wetsuits from Quintana Roo. This too defrayed the expense of racing.

In 1993, Lee gave me a special Christmas present: he hired a coach for me, Hank Lange. This came at the right moment as many of my triathlon rivals had coaches. I quickly discovered how helpful he was. Hank laid out the proper training for me after critiquing my techniques. For example, he filmed me underwater to improve my stroke; he also taped me on the bike, taking measurements and teaching me about proper cycling form—everything from maintaining an aerodynamic body to a fluid pedal stroke. The level of detail and nuance amazed me.

Hank even asked me to weigh myself before and after bike rides and runs, making sure that I wasn't getting dehydrated and was replenishing my fluids. He taught me about nutrition—a higher carbohydrate and lower fat diet was necessary to sustain my energy levels and protein was essential to fuel my muscles. He explained the importance of recovery, giving me a schedule of easier workouts interspersed between harder ones and a day here and there with no workout at all. He said the body needed rest in order to get stronger and described the benefits of rigorous training. Hank also reviewed my race schedules so that I'd be in peak shape for the key races, while scheduling "training" races in between to use as a gauge for my level of fitness. It was also terrific to have my own sounding board when things went wrong.

My husband trained too, though not nearly as intensely as I did. He worked for an insurance brokerage firm about twenty minutes from home in Syosset, Long Island, though mostly he did his workouts on weekends when we weren't traveling. While I raced to compete, Lee ran for the exercise and to stay in shape, and occasionally for the cold beer at the end of a race.

Lee and I constantly juggled our schedules to manage the training and the travel, which took us not just all over the US, but even to Europe. We traveled to places we'd never planned to visit—Terre Haute, Indiana; Lubbock, Texas; Rocket City, Alabama—and beautiful places we might never have seen—Saint Croix and Nice, France— had it not been the site of a race. We stayed with families who hosted us and we made an amazing array of new, enthusiastic, and welcoming friends. Triathlons created a special bond of togetherness between Lee and me, and I cherished the time we got to spend with each other as training partners and so much more. We were a team during these years of racing and training, anticipating each other's needs and supporting each other no matter what, in both good times and bad; as a family, and learning about commitment, camaraderie, perseverance, and trust.

But the schedules, the flying—a nightmare. The trips usually encompassed two or three nights, which also made them stressful— packing up the bikes and equipment, organizing childcare for the boys when they couldn't travel with us—and I never liked leaving the boys behind. I was a terrible flyer, worrying about what would happen if the plane crashed and who would care for our children. Of course, my stress also related to the pressure to race well. As I moved up the ladder, racing suddenly became a job, and the anxiety and the stress of meeting someone else's expectations—coach, sponsors, even family and friends—a steady corollary. I could see the downside to my passion for the sport, my competitive push to win. But this passion for triathlons and pushing the limits, and having to win, knowing I could win, also gave me confidence to face other life challenges.

As I thought over those long ago days, my mind kept turning to Lee who was now in the hospital. We had thrived on a vigorous athletic lifestyle, and if that was taken away, who would we become? And I couldn't give it up; I couldn't bear that thought and shoved it away. After all, that was no way for a determined and goal-oriented athlete to think. No, I knew I couldn't worry about something that hadn't been identified. What was the point in that? And if something was seriously wrong, we would tackle it and find a way to fix it, whatever it was.

I don't think I slept at all the night before Lee's bone marrow test. He and I had not yet spoken the one word that I knew haunted us both: cancer. You might think being an endurance athlete and having had to stare obstacles in the face routinely, I could have broached the subject with Lee. However, runners are human and fallible, too. In this case, I also refrained from talking about it in deference to Lee, because for him cancer was a huge fear.

When Lee was in high school, doctors diagnosed his father with colon cancer and he had to have a colostomy. He and Lee thought it'd been beaten. At age fifty, though, the cancer returned with a vengeance, and this time Lee's father lost the battle. His death at age fifty-three broke Lee's heart. Years later, tests showed that Lee's younger brother, at age forty-eight, also had colon cancer, and he died within the year. With both his father and brother dying so young, Lee had been diligent about getting an annual colonoscopy, but now as he approached fifty-four, I was quite sure that he feared the worst, not that he had colon cancer but that a cancer was surfacing elsewhere in his body and would kill him. I told myself I should wait for him to raise the topic. Anyway, the doctors knew his family history, and I assumed they would look for anything that pointed to cancer. Excuses, excuses!

On the Wednesday morning of that last week in Delray, I gave up on sleep around 5 a.m. I had my coffee, went for a run, then came back to the apartment and began cleaning furiously. I had to stay busy. A few times, I spoke to Lee in his hospital room. He had various doctors with different specialties stopping by, taking blood for assorted tests.

I pleaded with Lee to make sure he told each doctor who visited him everything that was worrisome. "Tell them you have no appetite for food or liquor. Tell them you've been waking up in the middle of the night with night sweats, your T-shirt soaking. Tell them your leg hurts and they need to check your hamstring. And tell them you have no sex drive"—something that was upsetting my husband a lot and that might get their attention.

It seemed like forever waiting to hear from Lee again. I couldn't eat, and I couldn't sit still. I should have been there.

At lunchtime, I wandered down to the beach, thinking that a good, strenuous walk along the ocean might help. I pretended Lee strode alongside me, although I was marching down the beach with much more vigor and speed than on our normal walks. Lee wouldn't have liked the pace one bit. As I forged ahead, I thought of all the questions I wanted to ask the doctors.

I was watching the time constantly, wondering why I hadn't heard from Lee. After being back in my chair on the beach for several minutes, my cell phone finally rang. I'd set it on the loudest ring so I wouldn't miss the call and nearly fell off the chair when the sound blasted through the air. Thank goodness it was Lee. He said the bone marrow test had been very painful but it was done. Now we had to wait for its result, and the results of the many other tests.

After Lee's call, I breathed more easily. He seemed much more relaxed and at ease than I was, undoubtedly relieved that testing was over. He seemed much more concerned, in fact, with trying to assure me that everything was going to be fine. He often told me I worried too much—but to me that came with being a wife and mother.

I turned to my computer and wrote the first of what became a regular group-email update, this one to the boys, my sisters, and several friends. Everyone wanted to know how things were proceeding with Lee, and this became the easiest way to fill them in.

January 27, 2010

Hi, everyone. Easier to send a group e-mail. Lee had his bone marrow test today at noon. Said it was pretty awful. Results from that will not be back till Friday or possibly later, but in the meantime, there may be some good news. The infectious disease doc saw him this morning and said that there are infections that he can get that are hard to fight because of the lack of his spleen. Something we had both sort of forgotten about. So that doc took more blood (if there is any left!!) and ran some tests. He also scheduled him for a cardio sonogram??? which he had at one today. The doctor just came back in and told him they found an infection in his mitral valve to his heart. Good news is they can treat that with antibiotics. They are giving him another IV with the antibiotic right now and hoping that will remedy his low red blood cell count. Not sure how long it takes to work, but he seems to be encouraged. They still have to continue with the other tests to make sure that is the cause of all this. He's hoping that will make him feel better because he certainly does not want to miss his opportunity to go back to college this weekend at UNC!!! Cryder, you will also be happy to know that he was finally allowed to eat something and just wolfed down a delicious turkey sandwich!! Your fave! Will let you know if there is any more to tell you, but maybe all our prayers are working!! Thanks to all of you.

xox

Early that evening, Lee called again with the official results from the cardio-sonogram that had been done shortly after the bone marrow test. They had solved the mystery! Although the results of the other tests still had not come in, the infectious disease doctor decided that Lee had an inflammation of the inner lining of his heart, a condition known as endocarditis. They would treat it with IV antibiotics through a port inserted in his arm to receive the medicine, but he said they would discharge him in the morning after checking his blood and heart again. Amazing how long it took to reach this conclusion, but thank goodness for that doctor!

Thursday promised to be a packed day, but even so I began it with a two-hour run—this was going to be my last long and warm run for a while. I also needed the time to think through many things before facing my day—this was my mental workout. Running was the best time for that. No outside distractions, just the sound of my feet hitting the ground. It was peaceful and solitary. I fully expected my legs to feel heavy after the stress of the previous few days, but I was pleasantly surprised that, with each step, my spirits began to lift and my pace increased. It helped knowing Lee was on his way to recovery.

The apartment that day had to be thoroughly cleaned for our renters, with all our special things tucked away in our "owner's closet." The refrigerator had to be emptied and washed, as did the food cupboards. The renters would be arriving in four days, on the first of February, and staying until the end of March. The day flew by as I focused on getting everything done before I had to leave early the next day. Lee and I talked several times. On an early call, he told me he wouldn't be discharged now until Friday because the doctors wanted to do another test to confirm the endocarditis. Unfortunately, those tests came back inconclusive later that day, so more tests were scheduled.

I truly felt horrible now. He needed me. And I worried about our plan to meet in Chapel Hill for Cryder's game. I was exhausted from my day, and even though I couldn't wait to put my head on the pillow, my mind still raced with the thought that I should have been with Lee at the hospital, because he had always been there for me.

I would never, in fact, have raced my first Ironman had Lee not been at my side at another race—Saint Anthony's Triathlon, in Saint Petersburg, Florida—that I entered in 1994 when I had just turned thirty-six.

Lee and I were both aware that the Saint Anthony's Triathlon was a qualifying race for the Ironman World Championship in Kona on the big island of Hawaii, but I had no intention of competing in an Ironman when I began training for Saint Anthony's. I knew it would be hard to get the Ironman slot while racing against such a very competitive age group, many of whom were vying for the position. Besides, competing in an Ironman event that consisted of a 2.4-mile swim, 112 miles of biking, and a full 26.2-mile marathon—in other words, double the swimming and biking distance I'd ever done—seemed far-fetched and beyond my reach. Unachievable. Did I say unachievable?

Lee had decided to run the race, too, and having him on the course always energized and cheered me, especially when we caught glimpses of each other on the out-and-back sections of the bike and run where we shared a thumbs-up or a shout of encouragement. Lee always joked that his motivation for competing was the post-race beer that organizers offered at the awards ceremony for a job well done.

As for me, well, my motivation was to win, and that early morning in Saint Petersburg, I'd run what I thought was close to a perfect race. Sometimes in a race, everything just seems to go as planned. I was able to get out front in my wave of swimmers and not waste a lot of energy fighting for space. My legs turned easily on the bike and with each stroke of the pedal I gained confidence. On the run, I seemed to fly by other competitors and ran strong over the finish line. An hour after my finish, my adrenaline was still pumping. Lee was enjoying his morning beer as we gathered in the open field with the other athletes awaiting the results and the awards to be announced.

If you won your age group, you also won a slot to Kona. We listened to the ceremony as victors squealed with delight, dashing to the stage to accept their certificate to Kona. Then I heard my name over the loud speaker. I'd won my age group and had beaten all but three of the pro women!

The announcer asked if I wanted the spot for Kona. Lee, surely encouraged by the beer, jumped from our spot on the grass and screamed, "She'll take it!" I stood speechless, my heart thumping. Seriously? As I hustled to the podium for my award, I couldn't wipe the smile from my face knowing that I had the go-ahead to accept this ultimate challenge: to become an Ironman!

The Ironman turned out to be a pivotal race not only for my career, but for what it taught me about life, as well as the physical strength it confirmed and the emotional strength it gave me. Tenacity, grit, and sheer determination. Sure, I had been racing for years, but this race would demand so much more of me, more than I would have ever imagined. It would require pushing the boundaries of pain and determination beyond what most would call impossible.

With the decision made, I now had six months to train to compete in the world championship of a distance I had never completed. Hawaii would be punishing: the heat and humidity, the terrain, biking through lava fields where the winds could be brutal and no trees to provide shade. But I also knew that I often raced better in such hot and humid conditions. I had learned much about training too. I knew that the training was the grueling, never-ending part; day in and day out, pulling myself out of bed and out the door, overcoming the fatigue and sore muscles while gaining mental stamina with each workout.

I had been working with my coach, Hank Lang, for nearly a year and trusted him to make the right decisions as I prepared for my first Ironman. Not only did he design the training routine, but he also kept me from second guessing myself. First and foremost, preparing for the Ironman meant stepping up the hours. I needed to fit 100-mile bike rides, endless laps in the pool, and 20-mile runs into a schedule that also included taking care of my two sons—now ten and seven—and of course paying attention to my husband. I trained four to seven hours a day, six days a week, building strength, stamina, and speed from that May until the race in October. The coach had me time my workouts—running, swimming, and biking—with the results telling him whether I was responding to the training or not. Some weeks were harder than others as we continued to increase the mileage in all three disciplines. Toward the end of the training, for three weeks in a row, I covered 15 miles of swimming, 300 miles of biking, and 80 miles of running. By the end of that period, I never wanted to see a bike again!

Then it was time to start my taper and cut back on the training, slowly reducing the mileage in each discipline by about ten to fifteen percent each week. The days I worked to keep my speed up remained intense, but reducing the mileage allowed my body to rebuild and to store the energy I would need on race day. I was amazed to discover how resilient my body could be, how it could bounce back and be even stronger after being put through such extreme exercise.

I wasn't Superwoman, that's for sure, though I made a huge effort to continue to meet my commitments as a mother and wife. Even when I was barely able to move after a workout, I'd force myself off my bike to kick the soccer ball with my son for a half hour. Most mornings, I dragged myself out of bed before the sun rose to get my training started while the rest of the family slept, made my way home to fix breakfast and get everyone out the door to start their days, then returned to finish my training before camp or school was over for the boys. In the meantime, I was trying to keep up with my new career as a coach and personal trainer. Time management was key, and I had to be flexible when things didn't go as planned—when the kids just wanted their mommy! I tried to remain upbeat and with a smile on my face, even when I was completely exhausted, in the hopes that Lee wouldn't tire of my training. We both felt plenty of tense moments, and I didn't blame him when he grew frustrated and wanted the whole thing over. He wanted his wife back!

Since it was a family effort—a sacrifice really—to get me in form for the race, Lee, Tim, and Cryder were determined to see me finish in Hawaii. Lee's father had been an American Airlines pilot, which made us, as family, still eligible to fly on standby passes, and that made the trip affordable for the four of us. I was to leave early Saturday morning a week before the race so I could arrive in Kona and have time to get used to the weather and familiarize myself with the course.

Best-laid plans don't always work, however. When I went to tuck Cryder into bed that Friday night and say good-bye before I left early the next morning, my usually self-reliant seven-year-old burst into tears. "Don't leave, Mommy!" he sobbed. I went back downstairs and told Lee: "Change of plans, Cryder's coming with me at 4:30 tomorrow morning." I had already packed his suitcase, so all Lee had to do was call Cryder's first-grade teacher on Monday and tell her Cryder would not be in school the next week.

Lee and Tim arrived as planned on Thursday night, exhausted from the travel but thrilled to be in Kona. And my mother, brother, and sister Kitty, also eager to witness the event, arrived late Friday night. My wonderful cheering squad was complete. I knew how lucky I was. The pressure was still great, but my guys—my family—were an amazing source of support.

The Ironman begins with a mass swim. There is extreme chaos as 1,500 people tread water all around you, waiting for the gun to go off. Then, at the starting horn, arms flail madly and legs kick everywhere. You feel as though you are in a fish tank in the center of a feeding frenzy.

When the race started that morning, I fought for room and somehow found a ribbon of space to begin swimming the 2.4 miles of the race. I got bumped and dunked, swum over, kicked, and pommeled. It was scary and intimidating, but I had to keep swimming no matter what. I kept telling myself: *Keep kicking, keep your arms moving. Go, go. When you make it to the bike, you'll be OK.*

After an hour of swimming, I emerged from the water, ripping off my overly tight goggles, a necessity to keep them from dislodging, and relieving the intense pressure around my eyes that had given me a massive headache. I was completely water-logged, lips swollen from the salt water, and disoriented and a little wobbly, but I quickly gained my land feet and raced through the transition. I threw on my helmet and glasses, stuck my feet in my cycling shoes, and adjusted the buckle on my bike pedal as I began the ride.

Somewhere behind me, on the way out of town, I could hear my family cheering for me. Their voices boosted my spirit and resolve— just what I needed to send me out on the next leg of the race.

The conditions on the road were something I'd never experienced. The lava fields looked like the moon—a very hot, windy, unfriendly moon. Biking 112 miles on the Kona coast is a true feat. You have plenty of company on the roads, but you have to keep your distance or get disqualified for "drafting," or riding in someone's wake. This is an individual sport—no help from anyone else is allowed. If you get a flat tire or have a mechanical problem, it's up to you to change the tire or make the repair, all while the clock is running. A handful of universal support crews travel the course offering to assist broken-down cyclists, but they are few and far between. Waiting for them to fix a problem can cost you precious time and knock you out of the competition.

At the halfway mark of the bike ride—mile 56—I checked my watch and saw that I was on target for the finish time my coach and I had projected. The race was going as we had planned, and I hoped I would also have enough energy to make it through the marathon. In a race like this, it was important not to look at the whole picture—that was too daunting. I needed to break it down into "doable" parts, efforts I felt my body could handle—a segment or a number of miles at a time. A mind game, to be sure, but an important one. It actually works.

As I approached town and the end of the bike ride, I had been in an aerodynamic position for a full 112 miles and about 5.5 hours, so long that my back felt as if a knife were sticking in it. I no longer wanted to be sitting on the horrible bike seat, with my rear end screaming at me to get off. *Ignore the pain*, I told myself. *Mind over matter*. Hundreds of people lined the streets. I stood up to pedal to try to unstiffen my legs for the run. I wasn't sure how my legs would carry my weight when I got off the bike, and I tried to prepare my muscles before the dismount.

I searched the crowd as I climbed the last hill, knowing Lee, the boys, and the rest of my family would be there. I rose out of my seat, pedaling hard, trying to look strong so they wouldn't worry. Again, a rush of adrenaline when I heard them yell. I can always hear Lee's voice over the din of a crowd. His distinctive words—"Way to go . . . You got it . . . Come on, Babe . . ."—still ring in my ears. There was less than a mile to go to my favorite part of the race: the run, my chance to shine. I could make up some time I'd lost in the swim and cycling segments, where I usually competed in the top twenty-five percent of the pack, but not out front.

Coming out of this second transition, I felt energized. I set my mind and my pace for the 26.2 miles. For the first few miles of the run, my legs felt unsteady, as though I were running on stiff boards. Slowly, my stride returned as I visualized myself running more powerfully and as my legs transitioned from the bike to the road.

I grabbed water and Gatorade at each stop I passed, trying to refuel what I had lost on the bike. Staying hydrated was critical. I had been mindful of that on the bike, making sure to drink from the bottles I carried with me, then tossing the empties to grab fresh bottles from the aid stations throughout the course. It was three o'clock in the afternoon, the hottest time of the day, but that couldn't matter. Now on the run, I finally started to feel really good, and I started to pass other women. The road was so hot that heat waves shimmered across it. Still, I kept my eyes focused ahead, searching for the next woman to pass.

At about mile 20, the effects of the long day began catching up to me. My strength started to wither. Now, I only passed people who were walking—they couldn't run, but they refused to give up. Their perseverance impressed and encouraged me; they were still going, so could I. Still, the march to the finish line suddenly seemed endless. In the past, whenever I started to falter in a race, I would begin a familiar conversation: *Come on, one foot in front of the other. Don't give up. Keep looking ahead.* This time, though, it would take a lot of talking, and setting ever smaller doable goals: make it to the next telephone pole, or the top of that hill.

With a little less than six miles to go, I set the goal of running from water stop to water stop. They were placed every mile. *Run to the water stops, come on. You can walk through the water stop, then run to the next.* It was a struggle. *Be strong,* I commanded myself. I knew that there was more at stake here.

Lee had brought a bike to Hawaii, too, so he could ride out on the run course and find me in a few places to cheer me on. He couldn't ride alongside me because that would be considered pacing and outside aid, but he could bike ahead of me and wait as I ran by him. No cars were allowed, so this was the only way he could cheer for me along the course. He appeared at various 3- to 5-mile intervals to give me a shout of encouragement. He knew well how I moved, and that day he could see I was faltering. Again, his encouraging words gave me strength.

"Come on, Babe, almost there. Keep it going. Only a few more miles to go." I had to make it. And I again began passing people who were running, which gave me a boost.

Coming back into town, I turned the corner to see Lee and the rest of my family halfway down the hill. They spotted me and began cheering wildly. "Almost there," Lee screamed. "Just a half mile to go!" Tim and Cryder were shouting, too: "Come on, Mom, you can do it!"

I took a deep breath and set my eyes on the finish line. It was just in front of me now, a beautiful sight. The finish line! As I passed under the Ironman banner, I looked up to see the clock. It read 10:22:43.

Lee stood on the other side of the finish line (he managed to get there somehow!) and proudly exclaimed, "You finished in the top twenty women! Awesome job!" I'd beaten several hundred women in this grueling competition! I'd come in nineteenth overall female and first in my age group (thirty-five to thirty-nine). Elated and exhausted, I tumbled into Lee's outstretched arms. That night I would celebrate with all my family.

In Hawaii, I had accomplished what I had never dreamed of a few years before, and I'd done it with my family's support, though mostly because of Lee and his belief in me. He'd known I was ready for this, or that I was at least ready to push myself both mentally and physically to succeed. And the Ironman race did confirm for me how powerful the mind, as well as the body, can be. Tell yourself you can do something you had thought impossible, and it's possible to make it happen. My mind was put to the test so many times in so many races, and whether I won or not, I learned that facing the challenge made me stronger. Also wiser. It taught me a discipline that would serve me well in facing the ups and downs of life: confront every challenge with a determination to defeat it.

I knew that having Lee at my side, understanding and encouraging, had helped me through all of my races and life's trials. And I knew, even in January, that I would draw on both the physical and emotional

strength that racing had taught me to guide us through whatever challenges faced us with Lee in the next months. Secretly, I hoped that the
endocarditis diagnosis would turn out to be accurate after all, and with
treatment Lee would be back to his old self in a few weeks, and we'd
be racing along together again, against the wind.

But deep down I knew we were in another race entirely.

9

Nurse McNicey Returns

That Friday in Delray, when Lee was in the hospital, I got up with the 5:15 a.m. alarm, which I'd set to allow time to get the sheets washed and back onto the bed, plus finish cleaning out the fridge and give a final sweep to the kitchen and bathroom and then one last run before I left. Since running in the dark was a bit too scary, I did these things first so the day would be brighter by the time I went out to run. After the cleaning and the run, I even had a chance to check emails one more time. I'm not sure why I had the energy to do all this—nerves?—for I certainly wasn't sleeping or eating well.

After a frantic morning, I arrived at the airport in West Palm an hour ahead of my noon flight, only to discover a weather alert. Snow was expected in Chapel Hill, where people don't handle snowstorms well at all. I was on Southwest Airlines because that airline had a connecting flight to Raleigh-Durham through Baltimore. This way, Lee would board the flight in Baltimore, and we'd travel to Raleigh-Durham together. A good plan, I had thought.

When I went to check in and saw the weather delay, I immediately phoned Cryder. If I checked my bags all the way to Raliegh-Durham, and got to Baltimore to find the flight canceled . . . good luck finding my bags again. It was already snowing in Chapel Hill and expected to continue throughout the day. The game was still scheduled to go on, but looking more and more questionable. I also called

Lee since we hadn't talked since early that morning. A very weary voice answered.

"Hi, I'm still in the hospital. Not sure if I am going to get out in time to make the flight."

"Oh, shoot. What's going on?" I didn't like the sound of that. Another full day of testing?

"I'm still waiting for the release from the doctors and for the port for the IV drip."

"Jeez, you're kidding. I'm so sorry," I said, feeling awful for him, and went on to explain about the weather and that I'd already been in touch with Cryder, who thought the game might not happen because of the predicted heavy snowfall. Lee and I decided I should cancel the trip to Durham and just fly to Baltimore instead. The Durham flight would most likely be canceled anyway, and I refused to go without Lee. If they rescheduled the game for Saturday, we could get up early and drive down. Neither of us wanted to miss one second of Cryder's last season of lacrosse, something that Lee had been looking forward to all week. I knew Lee felt really disappointed and, even more, was starting to feel trapped in the hospital. I had to get home.

As soon as I landed I called Lee, expecting to hear a happier voice because I figured he'd be home. Not the case—still in the hospital. This was getting ridiculous. I told him he was being a very good sport, though, and he said he expected to be getting out within the next thirty minutes. His car was still at the hospital, so I grabbed a cab home, hoping he would beat me there.

It was freezing cold when I opened the cab door in our driveway. It would take some time to acclimate to this temperature after the warmth of Delray. Lee still had not arrived home, so I went inside to reacquaint myself with my cold house. It was surprisingly intact after having been abandoned right after Christmas. I figured I had time to send a quick email before Lee got back so I could give him my full attention when he did walk in. I had become attached to my emails over the past several days, with so many family and friends wondering what was going on with Lee. But it was also time-consuming to reply to everyone. So I developed a single list of recipients, which seemed to be growing as more people wrote and asked for updates. I sent an email, and then waited and waited for Lee. In the meantime, I unpacked, straightened things, checked my emails and watched the clock some more. Where was he?

January 29, 2010

Hi everyone. Last I spoke you, they had diagnosed Lee with endocarditis. They followed up with another test yesterday morning, putting a tube down his esophagus to look at his heart hoping to confirm the bacterial infection on one his valves to his heart. Unfortunately, the test was inconclusive . . . so . . . they had taken some more blood samples to test for bacterial cultures. They could no longer assume it was endocarditis. He had to stay in the hospital again last night waiting for those cultures to come back, as well as the bone marrow sample that was due back this a.m. All the cultures did not allow for any definite conclusions. But the good news was the preliminary bone marrow test has come back negative. Phew! They still have to dig deeper on that to make sure there are no indications of any blood cancers, but so far so good. Right now he is getting more antibiotics through IV and is coming home this afternoon. They had to put a port in his arm so WE can hook up a bag of antibiotics every day for the next six weeks. So Nurse McNicey is back in action! Tim suggested an Absolut/grapefruit juice drip instead. Of course!!! As for now, because the bone marrow test was negative so far, they are going to treat him like it is endocarditis . . . all symptoms still point to that. But . . . he has to go back on Monday to check red blood cells and they may decide to do a liver biopsy. So please keep saying your prayers. Poor guy has had a rough week. Thanks to all of you for the calls and the concerns.

xoxox

Finally, at 5:30, I heard the garage door open and Lee's car come down the driveway. I met Lee at the door and noticed how he looked like someone had beaten him up. He fell into my arms, exhausted and relieved that I was home to take care of him. His hair was all over the place (funny but not surprising), and when he took off his coat and showed me his arm, it was bruised all the way from wrist to shoulder.

"What happened?"

"IVs," he said wearily.

Whoever inserted them clearly had had trouble. He showed me the port with a portable IV attached that looked like a small bowling ball. As the drip went into his arm, the ball would shrink. It seemed to work on suction and was actually fascinating. I would learn all about it, I figured, when the visiting nurse came on Saturday to give me instructions and explain my duties. (Though the endocarditis diagnosis remained inconclusive, the doctor had decided to continue the antibiotic, certain that Lee had an infection.)

As it turned out, Cryder's game took place as scheduled that evening, despite the snow. We were disappointed to miss his first game, but his girlfriend watched dutifully and texted us with regular updates and photos. She said it was crazy that they were playing; they had trouble finding the small white ball in the snowstorm, but the guys played well anyway and found what humor and fun they could as they slipped and slid about the field, something our boys used to love when they were young.

I got a chance to speak with Cryder briefly when he called after the game. He was pumped as always after a good win. Lee's birthday would coincide with the lacrosse game in Jacksonville the following weekend, so I reminded him not to forget and hoped he'd pick up a present for his dad. Lee treasured his Carolina Blue paraphernalia, and we teased him endlessly about it. But he could always use another item. That night was a better night for both of us. We were back together, and we felt the mystery was close to being solved.

In the morning, I snuck out of bed early, not wanting to wake my patient. We both needed our sleep, but there was much to do. And I treasured the early mornings. The house was quiet, and I had time to myself. I made coffee, hoping its heat would help keep my body warm for my morning run, and then I checked emails, grateful for one from Nini with calming advice about caring for Lee now that he was home. As I sipped my coffee, snow started to fall. The day before had been the coldest day of the winter, and the weather report now said today would be colder. Nonetheless, I bundled up and headed out the door for a freezing run. For the first few miles the cold air was burning my lungs and I felt as if I couldn't breathe, I persevered, continuing down my usual route, soon relishing the peacefulness of an early Saturday morning run; hardly any cars on winding country roads dusted with snow. Beautiful!

I thought about Lee again and again, about what a good man he was, and about how, through the years, on many of my long runs, he would come out and check on me. He loved and protected me. He knew my routes and where to find me. On hot days, he often tracked me down after a couple of hours and brought me a fresh bottle of water to replace the empty one on my water belt. And on one particularly memorable cold day in Baltimore—a nasty April day of sleet and rain in my final stretch of training just before another Boston Marathon—he again drove up alongside me. I was less than an hour from the end of my 20-mile run, and I was soaked and frozen. My hat was pulled so low over my forehead that I could barely see. I heard the car come from behind me and slow down. When it stopped, Lee rolled down the window and held up a dry pair of warm gloves.

"Thought you could use these," he said.

I was so happy to see him. "How did you find me?" I asked.

He just smiled. I stuck my frozen hands in through the window, and he pulled off my wet gloves and put on the dry pair. My fingers were too cold to work on their own.

"Are you sure you don't want to get in the car and ride home?"

He knew the answer as I shook my head. I had already considered taking a shortcut, but had decided not to give in. "No, I'm almost done, only forty-five minutes to go. Thanks. You're the best." He drove away, watching me in his rearview mirror, and I knew he'd be home waiting for me with a steaming cup of coffee.

That Saturday was no different. I came home from my frigid run with a frozen face to find Lee wrapped in his winter bathrobe, sipping his coffee and pouring me a very hot cup. He gave me a hug, sharing his body warmth. Again, it felt really good for both of us to be home.

The visiting nurse arrived midday, by which time a good dusting of snow had already collected on the ground. I was looking forward to this. I had nursed Lee through his hip replacements, and now I'd get to nurse him through this.

Nearly four years ago, when Lee discovered that he had to have both his hips replaced, he opted to do them at the same time so he wouldn't have to go through the whole process twice. He chose to have the surgery done in New York City. That was fine, except his other decision involved skipping a rehab facility and going home right after leaving the hospital. That, of course, meant I'd be taking care of him when he came home. All our friends and family thought that was extremely brave of Lee. They jokingly warned him: you are going to have Nurse Ratched taking care of you!

I did not think that was funny as I considered myself very patient and sympathetic. So when he was recovering at home, I treated him with care and ample kindness—bathing him, fetching things for him, taking him places when he couldn't drive or walk without a walker. I was a model patient-care nurse—even though it was a distinct change in our routine, first, to have him home all day, and second, that he wanted to be in the same room wherever I went.

At the time, I was a big fan of the TV medical drama *Grey's Anatomy* and its Dr. Derek "McDreamy" Shepherd, so, after a week of successfully and patiently taking care of Lee, I renamed myself "Nurse McNicey." My competitive side surfacing once again, I had to prove all my friends and family wrong: I was not Nurse Ratched. In retrospect, I think Lee would even agree with me that I was an outstanding nurse, except for one little incident when he claimed I tried to kill him.

One evening he'd gotten up in the middle of the night to use the bathroom. I heard the cane clunking along the floor into the dark hallway, and then—thud! I out of bed and found him lying on the floor. Well, actually on top of the suitcase I had left in the hallway between our bedroom and the bathroom. The one thing the doctors had warned him after his hip surgery was: "Whatever you do, don't fall." I leapt out of bed and stood over him with visions of hipbones protruding through his skin, afraid to check. I timidly felt his hips and found everything still in place. I sighed with relief. I couldn't lift him, though, so he had to crawl back to the bed, and with the two of us working at it, he got back on his feet. I am not sure if either of us slept well that night, but the next morning, reliving the whole episode, I started to laugh. The thud, my fear, his crawl—it was all too funny. Thankfully, Lee agreed. But he still likes to say I nearly killed him that night.

For Lee's care this time, we had already received several large boxes from Johns Hopkins Hospital, which we opened for the visiting nurse when she arrived mid morning. She began her instructions by explaining their contents. There were syringes, latex gloves, alcohol wipes, bandages, gauze, and more. The nurse described in detail how to change the IV and flush the line. It was a bit intimidating, but nothing I couldn't handle. She emphasized repeatedly how important it was to keep everything sterile. We both had to wear surgical masks when I changed the lines. I must admit that I thought this would be a nice challenge for McNicey.

It took a while for the nurse to go over everything. By the time she left, enough snow had accumulated that it needed to be shoveled. Wonderful—a chance for some exercise. Life was back to normal: me shoveling, Lee watching me shovel.

Over the next two days it continued to snow, and we learned that the endocarditis diagnosis was going under review, the reason being that the facts of Lee's illness were not stacking up neatly. Once again we waited, trying to stay hopeful.

By Monday, Lee had pretty much settled in on the sofa, distracted by the TV, while I continued shoveling snow. There was so much snow and only me to shovel. My arms felt as though they were stretched to the floor and ached with every movement. Every so often, I plunked down in front of the computer and sent off a few emails to friends and family. That was when I began my updates on Lee, using the subject line "McNicey Report." That morning, on the first day of February, we finally heard from one of the doctors and I shot off the first report.

February 1, 2010

Morning all. Woke up to 9 degrees and 6-plus inches of snow. Hooked our poor guy to his IV and went for a freezing cold run! Just came in from shoveling the driveway for a second time. Apparently our patient is not allowed to shovel. (I am thinking this is the same doctor that instructed me to shower with him for two weeks following his hip surgery to ensure that he wouldn't slip in the shower. Hmmmmm!)

Interesting news this a.m. Got a call from the infectious disease doc. (We call him Dr. House!) He has been so puzzled by our patient that he spent the night reading, trying to figure out what has infected Lee. Not sure if all of you heard Lee's rendition of finding a tick on his . . . well, let's just say I called him "ticky dicky" for a while! This past summer, after playing golf one day and searching for a few lost balls in the long grass along the course, he discovered this tick where it shouldn't be! He successfully retrieved it, took the tick to Patient First, where the nurses (after laughing at him in the back room) reported that it was an American dog tick . . . no worries.

Apparently there are all sorts of tick-related infections. The doctor thinks that he's been infected by a parasite called Babesia. It's carried by ticks and can infect people who are immune-compromised, which Lee is because he doesn't have a spleen. You can Google it and read about it.

So for all you wannabe docs who thought it was something like Lyme disease, you were right on track. He has to have another blood test tomorrow to confirm, but hopefully he won't have to suffer through the liver biopsy that had been planned. The treatment seems to be the same six-week IV treatment. So we will be traveling with IVs, syringes, saran wrap (for showering), and, of course, my best Nurse McNicey outfit!

So that's the good news: he'll be able to go to Cryder's college game next weekend. Thanks again to ALL of you for your e-mails and phone calls and concerns. Not to worry—he is in the hands of Nurse McNicey!!

xoxox

While Lee watched helplessly from the window, I continued my shoveling. At one point he came outside and picked up a shovel with his "good arm" and tried to push the snow using the shovel as a snow plow. The snow was too heavy for that and although I appreciated his trying to help, I shooed him back inside. He was supposed to be resting. By the end of the day, my whole being was exhausted, but more chores awaited me.

February 2, 2010

Well, I thought you all would enjoy an amusing little story about life with the McNicey's! After my day of waking up to changing Lee's IV line, a freezing cold run, then shoveling the driveway, then vacuuming and cleaning and laundry (remember, I have been away since right after X-mas . . . so you can imagine the state of the house . . . OK, OK, you don't feel sorry for me . . .) and most of all tending to my patient. I also had to fix two remote controls to two different

TVs which he managed to render dysfunctional. At 5 p.m., I diligently wrapped his arm with the IV port in saran wrap and tape as we were instructed so he could shower. I was taking a moment for myself, while he we showering . . . lying on the floor in the den, doing my evening stretching (my arms and back seemed a bit sore!!), when the phone rings. It was my longtime pal Weeder, whom I hadn't spoken to in a while and was catching up on the news about Lee, when I heard this string of four letter words streaming out of the bathroom with a desperate, "I need your help!" So I hung up on Weeder and raced to the bathroom where my darling patient had managed to CUT his extension line to his IV port! When he had gotten out of the shower, I called into him to see if he wanted help taking off the saran wrap. "No" he said, "Not yet." So he decided he would try to be "independent" and remove the wrap himself. Of course his vision is not so great anymore so he pulled out the scissors and tried to cut the saran wrap off his arm. He couldn't understand why it was "hard" to cut through the wrap and put a little extra pressure on the scissors and POP, there went the tube!! The one thing the nurse had told us was DO NOT expose the line to any kind of germs or infection. It had to be handled with surgical gloves, etc. Luckily, in our box of supplies from Hopkins was an extra extension hook up. So Nurse McNicey to the rescue . . . I put on my surgical gloves and reattached his line. All is good now. Needless to say, my patient is no longer allowed to handle scissors or a TV remote!! He will be at a loss without that remote, but that is the punishment he will have to endure!!

He had two more blood tests this morning and we will let you know the results when we hear. Poor guy has so many needle holes in his arms he's beginning to look like a heroin addict! Hope you all are well.

XOXO

∾ ∾ ∾

Our hope that the medical mystery had been solved was short-lived. After Lee underwent two more blood tests, we learned the good news and the bad news. All the tests for Babesia turned out to be negative. So the mystery remained exactly that. As for the good news, they would now remove the port from his arm because the IV antibiotics did not seem to be improving his health. Nurse McNicey was now in a semi-retirement, no longer handling the syringes, IVs, and showering responsibilities. Since Lee had managed to keep the port in place through the expected snowstorm tonight, there was no shoveling for him. But that was probably for the good because he continued to experience weakness, fatigue, chills, fevers, and a cough.

The doctor was convinced, though, that some sort of infection was plaguing Lee, and he was determined to find its source. The next step would be to "tag" the white blood cells in some type of radioactive procedure. White blood cells travel to the site of an infection and attack it, so by observing where the radioactively tagged blood cells went, the doctor would be able to find the infection. That appointment was scheduled for the following Thursday, so we would hopefully know more then.

Lee was beginning to feel very down and jokingly requested entertainment to cheer him up. But Nurse McNicey could only do so much. In the meantime, my goal was to stay positive and keep Lee's spirits up, just as Lee had always cheered me on and cheered me up, especially when I was down and out after a bad race.

In 1994, the US Triathlon Federation gave me the National Amateur of the Year award. I had just won my age group (females thirty-five to thirty-nine), and finished seventeenth overall female in my first Ironman World Championship. I had won a number of races and titles that year, and I now felt ready for a new challenge. I decided to up the ante and turn pro as a triathlete. In the triathlon world, you had to be ranked high enough as an amateur—basically, consistently winning your age group in national and world events—to be able to apply to the federation to race as a pro. Turning pro meant I would be eligible to collect prize money.

There was not much prize money in triathlons, certainly not like the hundreds of thousands, even millions, of dollars possible in golf or tennis tournaments because it was not as visible a sport and therefore not a money-maker for sponsors. In the smaller races you might win a hundred or two. In bigger races, like the Hawaii Ironman, you could win $25,000 for first place, and the top five or ten places usually also had a payout.

Another perk of turning professional was that pros were offered free race entries. The entry fees could get expensive—ranging from $35 for shorter races to $250 for the Ironman—and we paid double when both Lee and I entered a race. The savings from entry fees helped defray more of our costs, and that, plus my winnings, made sure money didn't stand in the way of racing.

Turning pro, however, also meant that, because triathlons usually start in waves, grouped by age or ability to make it a fair playing field, I would now be racing with all the pros in the women's open division. I was thirty-eight, and most of the pro women were much younger than that—not to mention obsessive—and many were single and without children. I was turning pro when women racers my age were setting their sights on retiring. But this was a challenge I wanted to meet, and so, despite the extra effort and the huge time commitment that would be required, I turned professional at the end of 1994 in time for the 1995 race season. Once again, my understanding family supported my decision. In fact they were excited about it.

As winter became spring in 1995, I trained with a greater purpose. I had decided my first pro race would be in April—Saint Anthony's Triathlon in Saint Petersburg, Florida. It was an Olympic distance race and the first big professional opener in the United States. My coach worked hard to prepare me for this jump in competition, and I worked hard to meet his expectations and be ready.

On race day, Mom and my sister Edie flew down to surprise me because Lee couldn't be there. But the race was a disaster. I came out of the swim far behind the lead women, and did even worse in the biking. I managed to gain some time back on the run, but I finished dead last among the pro women. I felt totally humiliated and embarrassed. Obviously I took the jump to pro status too lightly, thinking I was prepared to race against these faster women. Clearly I was not on their level.

My mother and sister were nothing but supportive and tried to lift my deflated ego. After a few hours, we joked about the big "L" (for loser) I felt I wore on my forehead. But deep inside I vowed this would not happen again. I now knew where I stood with these pro women, and I needed to train harder to reach their level. At home, Lee gave me more than a few pep talks to rally my spirit.

By June of that year, I was back finishing in the top five places in the local and regional races and feeling more confident. The hard work on improving my biking and swimming skills had paid off. More interval and strength training were a must. Still, my running was my forte, and I counted on that to pull ahead in the races whenever I fell behind on the bike. In a national event, I was still far from the podium, but I was thrilled I could keep up with some of the pro women and hopeful that I could learn from them and improve.

Through the next few years, I had some stellar finishes as a pro, and some disastrous ones. But I also discovered that the other pro women had similar experiences. The hard work just sometimes backfires when you overtrain and can't rebound in time to race or just simply have a bad day. After all, we are athletes, not machines. When it happened to me, I only worked harder to figure out what went wrong. Over and over again, I had learned to overcome, which is what I knew we needed to do with whatever test results came back for Lee. He could choose to give up or he could choose to regroup and fight. We knew which course we would take.

10

Sarcoma

Mother Nature must have been trying to give me a little zinger for abandoning my house for the past month. I woke early on Wednesday, February 3, braving the cold again for my much needed fix on the roads. I am not sure if it was the shoveling or the running, but I had now developed a cold, and cough too. When I run in cold temperatures, the adjustment my body has to make to deal with running outside in below freezing temperatures for an hour haunts me for the rest of the day. I get this chill that settles in and I can't seem to warm up for hours. I guess that is the nature of the beast, and maybe I should consider staying off the roads when its freezing and snowing, but that would not be me.

I have run for years in all kinds of weather. Some people set their watches by me, expecting me to be on my route when they're driving to work or taking the children to school. I am like the mailman; out on the roads no matter what. But, the thought of going back outside again, mid-morning, in below freezing temperatures, to shovel the new four to five inches that had fallen overnight, was not high on my list. This was not a nice welcome home!

I know Lee felt very badly not being able to help. He would have been right alongside me if he could, and he looked so down and out that I felt terrible for him. The one thing that gave him a lift was the visiting nurse, due mid-morning to remove the IV port as he no longer needed the line for the antibiotics. The downside was how discouraged we felt after another potential answer proved to be wrong. The looming liver biopsy was not anything either of us wanted to think about. But before that, they had to try tagging the white blood cells and hope to follow them to where this mysterious infection was hiding.

Thursday was frigid again, but I ran longer and faster than usual that morning, going over all of Lee's symptoms and tests and trying to come up with an explanation. Lee would be seeing his doctor that day at one o'clock, and I planned to go with him. I had enough of all this testing and I wanted to personally hear his explanations and give him a few of my own.

When we arrived that afternoon, the nurses greeted Lee like a good old friend. In my mind, they'd seen him too much lately. We waited for only a short while, thumbing through magazines until a nurse called us in. Accompanying Lee into the examining room felt awkward, making me think of taking the boys to their doctor's appointments when they were teens.

When the doctor walked in, the first thing I noticed was the long scar down the side of his neck. I knew better than to ask about it but assumed it was cancer related, and Lee later confirmed that. The doctor had had some strange cancerous tumor years ago, which made me think that he would be particularly alert to any cancer-related symptoms in Lee.

The doctor explained all the tests they had done so far and what they found and what they hadn't found. Finally, Lee swallowed hard and asked, "So we can rule out any cancer at this point, right?" I had no idea he was going to ask that question and felt my breath catch.

"Oh, yes, absolutely," the doctor said. "We've covered that."

I felt my body relax and exhaled a deep breath.

The doctor started to explain the next step, a test planned for the following week. They were going to "tag the white blood cells" and see where they traveled. Lee had already told me about this test and I knew the drill but listened politely. I couldn't sit still any longer, though, and said, "Doctor, I understand all these tests, but I'm really uncomfortable with this supposed hamstring tear you feel is the cause of the lump on his leg. I've been massaging it, as you suggested, but it's not getting better, and I think it has grown."

"Let's take a look," he said. "You don't mind dropping your pants with your wife here, do you?"

He obviously didn't know Lee very well.

"Be happy to!" Lee said, laughingly.

How embarrassing! The doctor examined his leg and then reached for his ruler, holding it along the lump. "Hmmm, you're right," he said. "This has gotten bigger." He narrowed his eyes in concentration. "I think we should get an MRI on this. The tear could have caused an abscess, and, with your compromised immune system, it could be causing all these symptoms."

Exactly! I was thinking. I knew this lump was the cause of his symptoms.

We went directly to the radiologist because the doctor wanted the MRI done before we left for Cryder's lacrosse game in Jacksonville, Florida, the next day. He said he'd call as soon as the results arrived.

Cryder's game on Saturday would be our first of the season, and we felt happy to be headed back to warm temperatures and, yes, palm trees! The weather forecast in Baltimore was for snow on Sunday and into Monday—a big storm was coming up from the south. Baltimore weather forecasters never seem to get it right, though, so I wasn't that concerned. Still, I thought I would outsmart Mother Nature and throw a snow shovel in the back of the car before we headed to the airport, just in case we flew back on Monday to find our car buried under a snow drift in long-term parking.

Many of the lacrosse team parents were traveling to Jacksonville for the weekend. We had planned on going with our good friends the Staines, Ron and Lauren, who lived near Annapolis. They had become our best travel buddies and great friends since meeting them through the team. We were all on the same flight and arrived in Jacksonville before noon.

Lee had a voice message waiting from his doctor. Yes, there was an abscess. The doctor was going to set up a biopsy for early next week. They would draw some of the fluid to see if this was the culprit, as I had suspected all along. Perhaps this time we were on the right track.

We had dinner plans that night with Ron and Lauren. On these trips, we really didn't get to see much of our boys as they had their schedule to follow, and we didn't want to be hovering parents. We seldom saw them before the game, and then the team bus would leave soon after the game. We usually managed a quick tailgate with the guys, load them up with food, and send them on their way, which would be a long way this time, back to Chapel Hill.

At Friday night's dinner, Lee offered to be the designated driver. He said he didn't mind because he wasn't really in the mood for a drink. Very unusual, I thought, because this was his birthday weekend. In fact, Lee usually claimed a full birthday week during which I was to shower him with gifts and attention.

Dinner seemed to take forever as I kept an eye on Lee. He was fading fast, and so was I. Instead of joining the usual UNC family late-night get-together, we ducked into bed on the early side. But our friends understood. Lauren, in fact, was a nurse, and I had been sharing all our test results with her, trying to get her opinion. Lee was not only tiring more easily as the days passed, he'd also lost weight. He wasn't exercising much as he had no energy, and he wasn't eating as much either. Nor was he drinking. The man who loved his occasional Bloody Mary and wine with dinner seemed to have no interest in any of that. Still, he looked great from the extra weight loss, so who was I to mention it.

Saturday morning, we all met again for brunch. I went for a run first while Lee, Ron, and Lauren all went for a long walk down the beach before we sat down to eat. Lee was physically exhausted when he came back, but mentally rejuvenated. Then the bad news: By the time we got to the game, the airlines were sending out snow cancellations. This time, of course, the weatherman had gotten it right.

It was good to see our boys on the field again. They were a bit rusty, but they still won—great for so early in the season. After the game, we only had about a half hour with the team before the bus left, barely time to hug Cryder and chat for a bit. Cryder hadn't seen Lee since the testing had started, and I could tell he noticed the weight loss. But there wasn't time to dwell on any concerns. One last hug for our son, and the bus was off.

Lucky that they were on the bus because many airports in the south were already closing down as the storm advanced. In the meantime, we parents madly tried to change flights. The prospect of getting on a flight earlier than Wednesday looked grim. So why not just rent a car and drive? I had already made the drive from Delray to Baltimore by myself, without stopping, and Jacksonville was three to four hours closer. We could make it in ten hours. With four of us traveling, it would be a piece of cake.

Lee was hesitant. The lump on the back of his leg had become so bothersome that he felt extremely uncomfortable sitting. But the thought of fighting our way back to Baltimore—being bumped around by the airlines and spending unknown amounts of time waiting for a flight—seemed daunting, especially with Lee feeling so tired. Driving looked like the best option. Unfortunately, with few snow-worthy cars to rent in Florida, we ended up in Ron's weekend rental, a Malibu. It was a four-door sedan with a decent amount of leg room in back, so Lauren and I—six-footers both—settled in for the entire trip home. We gave Lee the front seat, where the extra room might help him find a comfortable way to sit.

We'd gotten up at 4:30 a.m. on Sunday morning for our long journey back. Lee took some painkillers given to him by one of his UNC dad pals, something I would normally frown on. But he said the pain was such that he could not sit in a car for ten hours without some help.

Ron was a trooper, insisting on driving the whole way. He amusingly admitted he expected me to be like a caged hamster on an exercise wheel, running in place the whole way back—it's hard for me to sit still—but he didn't want the extra driving help. I do remember trying to push the accelerator several times from the back seat. Lauren and I made the best of the situation and entertained ourselves with story after story. By the end of the trip, there wasn't much we didn't know about each other. Lee slept a good deal of the way. The drugs may have been the reason, but it was a better way for him to travel.

The driving went well until just south of Washington DC, where snow had begun to accumulate and the roads were a disaster. It took us four hours to get to the Baltimore airport, where we'd left our cars, when it should have taken less than an hour. During the last two hours, our talking subsided as we all endured the slow pace and waited for the trip to end. Ron dropped Lee and me at our car, and we all memorialized the trip with a photo in front of the Malibu. Now another problem emerged: our car was buried. And the shovel in the back of the car would do us no good until I got through the two feet of snow that surrounded the car! The parking attendants said they had a Bobcat to help with snow removal, and it would be around to our car in about 30–45 minutes. I didn't think so! I was wearing loafers, a lightweight coat—and no gloves. I asked the parking attendant if he had a shovel, which he kindly handed over.

I started digging, determined to unbury our car and get us home. Lee sat in the bus watching helplessly. Eventually the driver felt guilty and offered some help. Together, after about fifteen minutes, we cleared the car enough to back out. The roads north of the airport were in much better shape, and we made it home faster than expected.

Our very kind neighbor had snow-blown a space just big enough for us to pull off the road into our driveway. We waded through snow up to our thighs to get to the front door. Neither of us had much of an appetite after our long journey. But we had arrived home just in time to catch the end of the Super Bowl, and then we collapsed into bed, Lee with thoughts of the unknown and tests that awaited him, and me with thoughts of . . . well, I knew what awaited me: more shoveling. I spent most of that next day digging us out.

Though Monday was Lee's birthday, we'd already celebrated in Jacksonville and he really wasn't in the mood for a big day, so opposite his normal exuberance for a week of pampering and attention. Instead, we had a quiet birthday dinner together.

Early Tuesday morning, on the ninth of February, we went to the hospital for Lee to have the abscess biopsied. While we sat in the hospital waiting room, a doctor friend from the pool where we swam walked by and saw us. He asked what we were doing, and Lee said he had an appointment. "Nothing serious, I hope," he said in a questioning tone. We laughed it off nervously and said no, just a follow-up to some tests. I wondered if he caught our lie.

When Lee finally settled into his curtained pre-op chamber, I joined him and we waited for his turn. They had to put him under, so he was all hooked up to an IV and dressed in his hospital gown. The doctor came in and pulled up a chair. He asked Lee to tell him about the lump; when he first noticed it, when it started to bother him, and so on. Lee described the whole thing, and the doctor listened carefully.

"OK," he said. "Well, I'm going to put a needle in and take some of the fluid and several samples of the tissue, as well."

Wait a minute. "What tissue?" I asked.

"Well, there's a mass there, and I have to take samples of the tissue, too."

Silence. I felt a lump grow in my throat and tears well in my eyes. I quickly looked up at the ceiling so I wouldn't cry. I was afraid to look at Lee. I could only imagine what was going through his mind. But, knowing that I was struggling to keep my composure, he took the reins.

"OK, I guess I'm all set. When will you have results?" he asked.

The doctor told us he would get the results to Lee's doctor by the end of the week. Then he slipped away and gave us the privacy we needed. I reached for Lee's hand and the tears came uncontrollably. I was terrified, but Lee was a rock and said, "I'm going to be OK. I promise you."

"Oh, God," I said. "They didn't tell us anything about a mass." I was afraid to say anything more. I had to get myself together for him. He reached for my hand and pulled me towards him, sharing his strength while I leaned into him, quietly crying.

The nurse came to wheel him away. I gave him a kiss and hugged him hard. "I love you" was all I could say.

"Love you, too," he responded. "It will be OK."

I put my head down to hide my tear-streaked face and wandered out into the hall, looking for a ladies' room where I could be alone. How could they have dropped that on us? Why hadn't Lee's doctor told us there was a mass? I felt angry and nervous and scared.

The procedure didn't take very long. Lee had only a light dose of anesthesia, so he recovered without much of a wait and we left for home. I kept my fears to myself and tried to be brave for him. At home, as always, numerous emails awaited me, but first I updated the boys, letting them know we were home and to give a call when they had time, though I tried to keep things upbeat and light.

And then I confronted the inevitable—more hours of snow shoveling. I would go out and shovel until I couldn't lift the snow anymore and then come in for a break. There was so much snow I could no longer find anywhere to throw it. Each shovelful had to be tossed over my shoulders atop the bank along the driveway that had grown to more than five feet high. My stubborn determination took over and I refused to let the snow win.

Eventually, I came inside for a break and flopped onto the sofa. Lee was sitting at the kitchen table when the phone rang. He picked it up. "Oh, hi, doctor." I watched his face for a sign, but he just kept saying "uh huh, uh huh, yup, okay, all right, yes, well, thank you." I was on the edge of my seat.

Lee hung up and looked at me for what seemed forever.

"That was the doctor," he said.

"Yes, I know."

"He said they did find quite a bit of fluid, and they're sending it to be tested." Then he hesitated. "But there's also a mass that could possibly be a sarcoma."

"A what?" I didn't like the sound of that word. "What is a sarcoma?"

"They won't know for sure until the tests come back. But it's some kind of soft-tissue mass."

I stopped breathing and felt sick. Three long strides and I was across the kitchen in his arms. I couldn't stop the tears. Lee struggled to be strong for both of us, but I think we each knew this meant trouble and that the worst was yet to come. We held onto each other for a while and then took a seat at the kitchen table next to each other, still holding hands. We spoke softly, trying to make sense of this latest news. The words did not come easily. I was trying to match Lee's courage.

"We shouldn't make assumptions," he said, "until we know for sure." With that he leaned over and gave me a kiss, then left the table.

I think he needed to be alone to think, to absorb what he had learned. He was also wiped out and needed sleep after a long morning at the hospital. My head spun. The doctor had said that we would have to wait until Friday morning for final results, and the possibility still existed that it was an infection instead of a soft-tissue growth.

As soon as Lee disappeared upstairs, I sat down at the computer and Googled "sarcoma." My hands felt sweaty as I read: Soft-tissue tumors were rare and tended to afflict children more than adults. But they were also hard to treat and didn't really respond to chemotherapy in that they didn't shrink. Then I panicked. Why had I read all this? I couldn't tell Lee what I had learned. I couldn't scare him with this information. I desperately wanted it to be something else. Lee was my whole world.

While I was busy researching sarcomas, the phone rang and made me jump. Cryder wanted to see if we had any news. My voice froze for a second, which was enough to tell him something was up. So I told him what we had learned. I tried to sound lighthearted, but he knew me better than that, and I could tell by his silence that he understood this could be serious. For his sake, I wished I could have told him in person, but for me it was a comfort just to hear his voice.

As soon as we hung up, I knew I needed to talk to Tim, too. But I didn't think I could put on a brave voice again to disguise my fears, so I sent him an email instead. I knew I should have called him, but I think I believed subconsciously that, if I downplayed what we feared, it might not happen.

February 9, 2010

Hey, wanted to let you know what's going on 'cause Cryder just called and I thought you should get the same info. The Dr. called this afternoon. They took samples of the fluid around the lump and from the lump itself. They have to wait till Friday a.m. to get results, but it could be either an infection (which is what we are hoping) or a soft tissue growth. As soon as we find out anything, we will let you know. Keep saying your prayers!!

Love you

xoxox

When I finished the email to Tim, the phone rang again, once more startling me. This time it was Mom. The minute I heard her voice, I burst into tears. She had been waiting to hear from us all day, too. Luckily, Lee was still upstairs napping as Mom did her best to comfort me.

I finally pulled myself together and explained what we had been told. She tried not to let me hear the worry in her voice. "Hang in there," she said "and we'll pray for the best." Lee was a strong young man, she reminded me, and he would be OK.

As Lee and I ate dinner that evening, I tried to keep the conversation light. I didn't want to think about what was happening in Lee's leg. He avoided the subject too. We just needed to wait. When we crawled into bed that night, we snuggled up to each other and held on tight. I was trying hard not to cry again, and I know he was, too.

He quietly whispered, "When you hugged me today after the doctor called, you were hugging me like you would never let me go."

"I know, and I'm not going to let you go." I was silent for a minute and then managed to add in a shaky voice, "You are not going anywhere without me. Got it?"

I could hear him swallow hard. No need to say more.

Lee rolled around all night, while I awoke several times and stared at the dark ceiling, my eyes wet with tears. I knew I'd have to reach deep, like I had in the Ironman, when I'd made it through the choppy dark blue waters off the coast of Kona, the excruciating hours on a bike, and the hills on the marathon course. I had gotten through that and I could get through this, too. I told myself I'd do better in the morning. I just simply had to be in stronger for Lee.

11

Lee and Lee

I was seventeen years old and a senior in boarding school when I met Lee. It was in December of 1975, and my sister Kitty was "coming out" at the New York City Cotillion Ball at the Plaza. My sister Edie had invited me to go with her to another party in Manhattan the same night. We were all meeting at my father's apartment in the city for a drink before Kitty's event. She had two escorts for the ball, both of them joining us at Dad's apartment. Lee was one of those escorts.

I had met Kitty's friend Dobbs, the other escort, but not Lee. Kitty had become friends with them in her first year of college up in New Hampshire. I'd heard her speak about both Dobbs and Lee many times and knew she had a big crush on Lee.

We arrived at Dad's to find Kitty looking beautiful in a long white evening gown. Edie and I also wore long dresses for our party, and all the parents—my father and stepmother and my mother and stepfather—were in formal dress, too. We were only waiting for Kitty's escorts to arrive, who were late. Finally, the doorbell rang and in walked Dobbs and Lee. My eyes were drawn to Lee immediately. He was a bit taller than me with wavy dark hair and gorgeous Italian skin. He had a gap in his front teeth like Lauren Hutton and a brilliant smile. Dressed in black tie and tails, he looked stunning. But he was Kitty's date, so hands off.

With five sisters so close in age, we all knew the rule: no stealing another's boyfriend. Over the years, at times, we broke that rule. Not intentionally, of course, but it happened. The joke was: never bring a boyfriend home. You can only imagine some of our guy friends' reactions when we invited them over and they found four other sisters in the house, sometimes seven when our stepsisters were in town, all within five years of each other.

The night of the Cotillion, we only stayed at Dad's apartment for a short while before we all had to leave. There was hardly time to have a conversation. I was shy around men then and tended to let my sisters do most of the talking. Kitty was whisked off in a limo with her escorts while Edie and I hailed a taxi to our party. My parents and stepparents were having their own dinner first and meeting Kitty at the Plaza Hotel later in the evening. Before we parted ways, Mom had given me the option of returning to Long Island with her and Jack. Knowing Edie tended to stay out into the wee hours of the morning, Mom told me that if I wanted a ride home, I had to be in the lobby of the Plaza by midnight. Just like Cinderella.

By eleven or so, I'd wearied of Edie's party. Everyone there was college age, and I wasn't enjoying myself. I decided to leave, knowing it might take a while to flag a cab. I arrived at the Plaza twenty minutes early. I knew the ball was in full swing a few floors up, but didn't feel brave enough to wander into the event uninvited. The lobby of the Plaza was virtually empty.

Then I heard a commotion. A flamboyantly dressed man was coming out of a bar followed by a posse of men and women; he was making a lot of noise and waving his arms all over the place as he strutted past me, laughing and swaying. I looked again and . . . it was Paul Lynde. I used to watch him on *Hollywood Squares*. He was ridiculously funny.

Then a voice from behind me said, "Hey, are you lost, little girl?" I turned around, and there stood Lee, smiling and looking like a star himself in his black tie and tails. Words refused to come. I felt horribly tongue-tied.

"What are you doing here?" he asked.

All I could say was, "Did you just see Paul Lynde?"

What an idiot—why was I so flustered? I told him I had to be in the lobby by midnight to get a ride home with Mom. He said he'd come down to the lobby to buy a pack of cigarettes—lucky for me!—and then he invited me to go up to the ball with him to find my mother there.

"Are you sure it's OK if I go?" I asked.

"Sure, you're with me."

I would fit in with my long white gown, so I followed him to the elevator and chatted nervously. He was still smiling. I was mesmerized. Then the elevator stopped and the doors opened onto a spectacular ballroom, the walls covered in mirrors. Huge crystal chandeliers hung from the ceilings, and in front of me, everywhere, beautiful young women in white gowns danced with men in their black tuxedos. Everything sparkled. Lee reached for my hand and led me toward the ballroom.

"Would you like to dance?" he asked.

"Oh, um, I, ah, sure," I stammered, "if you think it's OK."

He led me onto the dance floor. I reached up to his shoulder while he put his hand around my waist and rested it on my back. I was breathless as we danced. Then, over his shoulder, I saw Kitty, daggers in her eyes. Uh oh!

The dance was ending anyway, and I told him that I had spotted Kitty and that we'd better find her and my parents. I had to go. The Cinderella thing—it was midnight. I thanked Lee for the dance and for delivering me to my parents. I said good night to Kitty, who wasn't very friendly at this point, and we left. That was that, I thought. I'd never see my Prince Charming again. He belonged to Kitty.

After Christmas vacation, I returned to boarding school in Maryland for my final semester there. Although I thought about Lee and would listen carefully when Kitty spoke of him, our paths did not cross again for nine months.

At the beginning of September, I was attending a small college in Boston. I hated the school and felt miserable. I think I cried for a week straight after Mom dropped me off. Kitty was returning to her small college in New Hampshire, where a year earlier she had met Lee and Dobbs. Since her classes didn't start until a week or so after mine she asked if I wanted her to visit on a Friday night on her way up to her school. "Yes, please," I said. I was so lonely.

When it was time for her to leave on Saturday, she suggested I come with her to New Hampshire. We could both take the Greyhound bus up from Boston, and she would put me back on the bus Sunday night. So I went.

We made it to her college town by dusk and stored our bags in the apartment she was renting with friends. The first place she wanted to show me was the fraternity house where all her friends would be. We wandered down a small street and then along a dirt path lined with pine trees. The fraternity house looked like a replica of *Animal House*. Yuck! As we approached, two guys came out the door.

"Hi, Kath," said one—it was Dobbs, and the other was Lee. My heart started to race. That same smile, and now he had a summer tan. I told myself to act cool or Kitty would surely slug me. It hadn't occurred to me we might run into Lee. Only Dobbs went to school there; Lee attended Nathaniel Hawthorne, a school a few towns over.

We talked for a short while and then left. Kitty had to organize her apartment, and we had to buy food. But before we left, Kitty turned to Lee and asked if he could possibly entertain me tomorrow morning. She had to go register for classes and so did Dobbs and all their friends. But Lee was free because his classes started later.

"Sure," he said and agreed to meet me by ten.

My face was burning red, but I tried not to show my excitement. It surprised me that Kitty had arranged this, but she worried about me and knew how miserable I had been in Boston. She didn't want to leave me sitting in her apartment for hours. And perhaps she had forgotten about our dance last December.

The next morning Lee arrived on time. It was a sunny and warm day for New Hampshire. He said he'd give me a tour of the campus, so we walked and walked and walked. The campus was beautiful, with streams and trees and old ivy-covered brick buildings. He even walked me through a rickety covered bridge. We talked about everything that popped into our heads, although I don't recall the specifics, only that I was very enamored of him. The hours flew by and we met up with Kitty again. I thanked him for entertaining me, but I didn't want him to leave. I had a feeling he didn't want to go either. This time I sensed that maybe we would see each other again.

Over the next few weeks, Lee and Dobbs came down for visits in Boston. They knew several girls who went to my college and, supposedly, came to visit them. Lee was very popular! I did my best not to get jealous and kept telling myself we were just friends. But we found ourselves spending more and more time together. I could talk to him about anything. After I confided in him that I couldn't seem to find the right guy, we even discussed boyfriends. He assured me he would help me find the right man.

December, meanwhile, was fast approaching, and this was my year to attend the Cotillion in New York City. Since I was not dating anyone, I asked my new best friends, Dobbs and Lee, to be my escorts. After all, they already knew the drill.

Over Thanksgiving weekend, my sisters and I gathered at home from our various boarding schools and colleges. Only a few weeks before the Cotillion, Dobbs and Lee decided to make a road trip from New Jersey, where they both lived, to visit Kitty (and maybe me) on Long Island. The notion secretly thrilled me. I knew Kitty still had her eye on him, but after a year of friendship she also seemed to know that friendship was going to be as far as their relationship would go. Still, I was sensitive to Kitty's feelings as it was obvious to others that something was brewing between Lee and me.

By the end of Saturday night, when we were all heading off to sleep, I found myself alone with Lee. I walked him to the back of the house to show him the bedroom where he could sleep. My palms were so sweaty and my stomach was turning. "Well, this is it," I said and as I turned to say goodnight, he was right behind me, catching me off guard. He pulled me towards him and timidly kissed me. My head spun and my knees felt weak. I didn't know what to do so I smiled and said good night. It was a secret kiss—our secret.

That December, the Cotillion was even more magical. This time when I danced with Lee on that elegant dance floor, we fell in love. I was only eighteen years old and Lee was twenty, but from that moment on we saw only each other. Lee transferred down to Boston University in his last year of college so we no longer had to do the commute back and forth to New Hampshire. On the day after Valentine's Day in my senior year, Lee asked me to marry him, to be his Valentine for life. Of course I would, there would be no other. I had found the love of my life.

12

It's Cancer

On the day after the biopsy, Lee and I tried to stay busy. He went to work, and I called him several times during the day to ask, "Any news yet?" Nothing. I made the mistake of reading more about sarcomas while I waited. I had the computer on when I heard Lee opening the door for his midday nap. I quickly closed the screen, but I had just read some awful stuff. My eyes were red from crying. I needed to talk to someone, so I grabbed my phone, told Lee I had to run to the grocery store, which was only two minutes from our house, and disappeared out the door. I parked in the back of the lot and called my parents' house. My stepfather, Jack, answered.

"Hey, Kiddo."

I plunged right in. "Jack, I'm so scared," I confided. "I've been reading all this awful stuff about sarcomas and I'm so afraid that's what Lee's lump is. I don't know what to do."

"Listen, Kiddo," he said, "Lee's a healthy guy and way too young to have something like this. There are all sorts of things it could be. Don't panic. It's going to be OK. Let us know if there's anything we can do. We're right here."

Just to hear his voice and have his reassurance comforted me. It was probably good that Mom didn't answer the phone because I'm sure I would have just started sobbing again. With her I abandoned all need to be stoic; mothers allow their children to do that. But Thursday morning I woke early and found a worried email from my mother, sending me love and good thoughts. I answered her immediately.

February 11, 2010

Haven't been able to write a follow-up to everyone with the latest test results. I'm so worried that I can't bring myself to write. Hoping we will find out some news today.

Couldn't really talk about his situation openly yesterday because Lee was here and I don't want him to know how scared I feel. I Googled sarcoma and if that's what it is then I'm terrified. I know he is too. Woke up throughout the night saying long prayers. Thanks for the support and calls. Need it!!

I shoveled the whole driveway three times and am exhausted. Eighteen inches of new snow and nowhere to put it anymore. Lee is going to the office in the afternoon so will try you later today. Hope you all didn't get the same amount of snow we did!

xoxox

Thursday came and went with no word from the doctors. And on Friday, Lee went off to the office while I readied us for our drive down to Chapel Hill for another lacrosse weekend. I planned to pick him up at noon.

I went for my usual run in the morning. This helped me clear my head, which I needed more than ever. Somehow, answers to my questions came more readily when I ran. It was also uninterrupted time—a kind of physical meditation, in which mind, body, and soul united in the rhythm of running. The years of training and racing felt like a blessing now and I was grateful for the outlet.

Back home, I raced around the house, straightening up and packing the car. It was about eleven when the phone rang. It was Lee, making sure I was all set to pick him up at noon.

"Right on schedule," I said.

He was quiet for a minute, and then said, "The doctor just called."

My body tensed as I waited to hear what he'd said.

"The tests came back." Then silence.

"OK."

"It is a sarcoma."

My hand struck the desktop and tears sprang to my eyes. I couldn't speak; I didn't know what to say. My world collapsed around me.

"Hello?" he said. "You there?"

I closed my eyes tight and tried to control my voice. "Yes, I'm sorry. Are you OK?"

"I'm OK. I'll tell you what he said when you get here."

"I'm leaving right now. I'll be there in a few. I love you."

He hung up and I put my head on the desk and wept. This can't be happening. Not to Lee. I just knew it was his leg, and I grew angry at the doctor. Why had he told Lee over the phone when he was alone at his office? He could have at least told me first, but I knew what was really happening. I was redirecting my fears into anger. I had to get down there as fast as I could. First, I had to call Mom.

She picked up right away, as if she'd known I would be calling at that moment. All I could manage was a shaky "Mom." My sobbing burst forth then, and without any additional words she knew. Though devastated, she did her best to once again assure me that Lee, otherwise healthy and strong, would fight through this. And she added, "We still don't know what kind of sarcoma it is, so don't jump to conclusions." She said I had to be strong for Lee and not show him how worried I felt. She was right; I had to pull myself together. Hopefully we'd caught the cancer in the beginning stages.

I drove madly to Lee's office and waited outside in the car. A moment later, he appeared at the front step. A slow smile crawled onto his face as he waved and walked toward me. He seemed dazed. I leapt from the car and threw my arms around him. The whole situation felt better already.

In the car, I listened to Lee recount the conversation as we drove off toward Chapel Hill. A soft tissue mass, the doctor said, right at the attachment of his hamstring. He thought it was only in stage one or two, and he had already put in a call to the best doctor at Johns Hopkins to deal with this, a Dr. Frank Frassica, the head of the orthopedic surgery department. Lee said his doctor ended their conversation saying he would pray for him. I couldn't decide if that felt comforting or not.

Lee had also made a call to Dr. Ben Carson, a well-known, highly regarded neurosurgeon at Hopkins. Lee had served on the board of his charity, the Carson Foundation, for the past five years, and "Dr. Ben" was a friend. He said he'd make some calls immediately and get Lee in to see Dr. Frassica as soon as possible. His office called later that day to say Lee had an appointment first thing Tuesday morning. It was Presidents' Day Weekend, and Dr. Frassica was off on Monday

I tried to keep a level head as we reviewed all the information. Lee somehow remembered that my stepsister Leigh had had a cancerous lump in her leg removed a few years earlier. He remembered it being a sarcoma. Lee can remember the strangest facts—it's his dream to be on *Jeopardy* one day.

We called Leigh and, yes, she'd had a sarcoma. Hers had been a small lump in her thigh, and she opted to have the lump removed instead of going through chemotherapy. She said she had had no problems since. Good news. Maybe Lee's would also be just a simple procedure. They'll just go in, remove it, and that will be that.

We had a five-hour drive ahead of us to Chapel Hill. After talking to Leigh, I felt a little more confident that I could handle talking about it now, so we decided to call Tim. We thought it was better to wait until after the game on Saturday to tell Cryder. No need to distract him.

Tim remained quiet when we explained the results. I imagine it frightened him to hear the word "cancer," especially when we had no idea what would be involved in coping with it. After he'd asked numerous questions, he reassured us that he would be by his dad's side no matter what, reassuring me that Dad was a strong man and he had all of us to stand by him. Tim, being the older son, was fiercely protective of not only his younger brother but of me as well, and I knew I could rely on his strength. It also comforted me to hear how well he'd handled the news, though I'm sure he was as frightened as we were.

Lee and I spent the car ride mostly lost in our own thoughts. Occasionally, we dove into a conversation, distracting ourselves from what we were brooding about, but then we lapsed into silence again, the fear of cancer and the future surrounding us.

I thought a lot about Lee on that trip, and how truly physically able he was, as Mom and Jack kept reminding me. I was grasping, I'm sure, at this thought in hopes that his basic strength would help him through this. He had, after all, spent many years racing right alongside me in marathons and triathlons. And once, in his mid-forties, he had done this crazy mountain race in New York State called "The Survival of the Shawangunks." I had already committed to another race that weekend when a friend of his enticed him to join a group heading up to "The Gunks," about eighty miles north of Manhattan and just west of the Hudson River. The race began with a 30-mile bike ride, followed by a 4.5-mile run, then a 1.1-mile swim, then a 5.5-mile run, then another ½-mile swim, followed by another 8-mile run, then another ½-mile swim, ending with a very steep .7-mile run to a peak where a lookout tower was perched. This was all done on trails (except for the biking portion) around several lakes with freezing cold water. Suffice it to say, I was quite happy to be busy that weekend.

During the swims, you had to either strap your shoes to a belt around your waist or keep them on while you swam, which is really hard to do, but this was a point-to-point race with nowhere to pick up shoes or equipment as you followed the trail. When he got out of the water at the last lake to make his final run up the trail, Lee's legs cramped so badly that he fell to the ground. There were volunteers helping people out of the water, and they immediately tended to him, vigorously rubbing his legs to stop the spasm. He welcomed their help for a few minutes and then insisted that he wanted to get up and continue. The pain was crippling, he later told me, but he willed it away and forced himself to make the final run to the top of the peak, using his mind to shut out the pain. I was so proud of his effort and thrilled for him when he placed in his age group. Though unable to see him get his award at the event, I prominently displayed his plaque at home.

He may not have raced in years, but the physical and mental training he endured for that and so many other races was embedded in him, as it was in me. He would now have to rely on that physical and mental memory to renew his strong will to fight. He would have to survive "The Gunks" again.

When we arrived in Chapel Hill, Lee's mood visibly improved. We had so looked forward to seeing Cryder, his friends, and all our UNC family. When we ran into our friends, Lauren and Ron, they quietly pulled me aside and asked if there was any news. I told a little white lie and said no, because we wanted to tell Cryder before sharing this with anyone else.

After the game on Saturday, we went over to pick up Cryder for dinner. It was tough to get him alone after a game because all the guys had just this one night to blow off some steam. The rest of the week was dedicated to practice, and no nights out. But that night we managed to pull Cryder away and into the car. He was in the front, next to Lee, and I was in the back, wishing I could prepare him for what was coming. Cryder faced Lee; I could see the side of his face and I watched his expression as Lee told him the news. Cryder tried hard to be stoic. I wanted to reach out and hug him and tell him it was all going to be OK, but I forced myself to match Lee's calm as I watched Cryder deal with the pain and fear. Lee even tried to be lighthearted, I think both for his sake and Cryder's. He told Cryder that he had an appointment first thing on Tuesday and that we were going to have the doctors "go in and take that sucker out." Cryder put forth his best smile and agreed everything would be fine. But I could see the worry in his eyes.

Over the years, both Tim and Cryder had experienced the strong mindset needed to overcome tremendous physical obstacles as they watched us from the sidelines and at times saw us struggle to cross finish lines. Cryder knew the hurdles his father had conquered in the past, and deep down I think he remembered the determination he'd seen in his old man. It still had to be there, without a doubt.

The next morning we woke up early to get on the road and be home around lunchtime. Lee slept a good part of the ride home, and while I drove, my mind raced off in many directions as I tried to justify what was happening and figure out how to fix it. I could think of no solutions yet. All I could do was try to manage what I could control, which was how I responded. I remained positive that Lee would be OK and I tried to create fail-safes for my boys, asking friends to keep an eye on them, making sure they were being cared for when I couldn't be there.

13

We Will Beat This!

The day had finally arrived to meet with Dr. Frassica, the orthopedic surgeon, at the Johns Hopkins Medical Center. We were lost in our own thoughts as we approached the massive structure.

We arrived fifteen minutes early for our eight o'clock appointment. Lee and I both felt anxious and nervous; it seemed as if this surgeon held our fate in his hands. He gave us a warm welcome and then indicated we should seat ourselves at his conference table.

He had obviously done his homework on both of us as he continued speaking, expressing his interest in the physical and mental endurance required in the challenges posed by marathons and Ironman triathlons. I wondered why he was raising this topic, and although confused because we were not here to talk about me, I went along with the conversation. It was only later when I had time to think about the strength it took to compete in such events that I understood his reason for reminding me of my will to beat the odds. A little more small talk, and then it was time to get down to business. His focus then turned to Lee.

Again, Lee was asked to review the past couple of weeks and all the tests he'd had. The doctor wanted to know about the biopsy and how it had been performed. This was important, he said, because sarcomas, if disturbed, can break off cells that travel and plant themselves elsewhere. It was important that the biopsy was done with a needle and not a knife. The first place the cells tend to travel, he said, is the lungs, which would not be good. Thankfully, Greater Baltimore Medical Center had performed the biopsy the right way.

He went on to explain how rare sarcomas were, but he emphasized that this was his specialty. This knowledge provided some relief for both Lee and I—at least we were with the best. He pulled out a pad of paper and began to explain how sarcomas developed. First, he wrote down the size of Lee's tumor in inches: 9.8 x 5.1 x 5.3. That meant little to me because I had no idea if that was considered large or small. This was all new to us.

Dr. Frassica then started to explain the three grades of a sarcoma: 1, 2, 3, or low, medium, and high, respectively. We watched as he wrote all this down, and I wondered why we were discussing all three stages. Lee's doctor had already told us that his was a low-grade sarcoma, probably a 1, possibly a 2. But we listened carefully and gave him his chance to explain the different stages.

When he finished providing these details, his pen moved slowly across the page and stopped above the words "3 High." He circled this as he said, "This is what you have." His pen seemed to move in slow motion. My eyes were fixed on that paper. Lee had gone still. I stared at the circle. Then the paper started to blur as my eyes welled up. I searched for Lee's hand again, and once I found it, I squeezed hard. *Oh, God, please let this be a dream.* No one said anything until the doctor turned to me, put his hand over mine, and said, "Are you OK?"

"Yes, sorry. I'm fine." With my other hand, I squeezed Lee's hand tighter. *Be brave. Don't show him you're scared. He needs you.*

Lee took charge. He could see that I was fighting for control and he wanted to make this easier for me.

"OK. So what's next?" he asked, nodding his head and accepting what he had come to learn.

Dr. Frassica then explained the best way to treat these sarcomas. I listened as best I could, willing my head to clear and my mind to focus, just as I had so many times when I was in a tight spot in a race struggling to maintain control. I needed to remember what the doctor was saying. Then I heard "chemotherapy," which I hadn't thought would be involved.

Again, he wrote as he explained, probably knowing that we were only able to process half of all he said and would need to refer to the notes later. "There will be a series of steps," he said. Lee would spend three to four days in the hospital getting chemo, two days off, followed by eleven days of radiation and then five or so days of rest to regain his strength. After the first series, he would have to repeat the routine two more times—a grueling process.

The chemo, we learned, wouldn't help shrink the tumor, but it would work to deaden the area around it so that the surgeon would need to remove less of the surrounding tissue. After the three sets of treatment, Lee would rest for two to three weeks before surgery. He was in for a fight.

Dr. Frassica had already arranged for us to meet his young protégé, Dr. Attar, who would be our surgeon. We were also to meet with the rest of his team. The chemotherapist was alerted, as well as the radiologist, who happened to be Dr. Frassica's wife.

We gathered ourselves and thanked Dr. Frassica. Again, he thoughtfully asked me if I was OK. He led us out of his office into the lobby with all the portraits. I made a comment about the portraits and said maybe one day his would be hanging here. His reply was light-hearted: "I hope not too soon."

"Why not?" I said without thinking.

"Because these men are all dead!" he responded with a smile.

He gave us his card and told us not to hesitate if we needed anything at all, and he headed us down the hallway for our meeting with Dr. Attar. We were ushered into an examining room and asked to wait there for the doctor. As soon as the door closed, we turned to each other and, as would be the case again and again over the ensuing months, collapsed into each other's arms.

"I love you," I said, my voice trembling. Lee couldn't speak. I knew what he was thinking, and I held him tighter. "We will get through this," I said. "You are not going anywhere. Do you hear me?"

He was shaking and trying to hold back his own tears. *OK, we need to pull ourselves together*, I thought. The doctor was going to walk in at any minute. We sat in small armchairs next to each other, again grasping each other's hand, and waited in silence.

A knock on the door and in walked this seemingly very young man. He was incredibly polite and had a wonderfully warm smile. He introduced himself as Dr. Attar and told us he used to practice in Chicago but had been working with Dr. Frassica for several years. He asked if Lee would mind showing him his leg so he could examine the lump. He then went over the same information as Dr. Frassica and explained his role. Though everything sounded familiar, I felt like I was watching and listening from a distance. It seemed terribly surreal. Could this really be happening to us? Lee appeared brave, though I could only imagine what he felt.

Dr. Attar promised he would do whatever needed to be done to get that tumor out, and we believed him. From there, we were sent to another section of the hospital to meet with the chemotherapists. As we traveled the halls, I tried not to stare at the hairless patients with masks over their noses and mouths. I felt we were invading their world, though soon it would be our world, too. I could sense Lee feeling similar emotions. How I wished I could do something to comfort him. I clutched his hand and gave it a good squeeze. He squeezed back, letting me know he was coping.

We met with the chemotherapist, quite young and very pregnant, who told us that her baby was due at any moment. This meant she would not be able to see Lee through the whole process—unfortunate because we really liked her—but she'd get him started and leave him in good hands. Again, more explanations and more examining. Then more blood work.

The hospital staff shuffled us from office to office, from one waiting room to the next. It was an overwhelming and exhausting experience. We'd anticipated a short appointment during which we would set up a time for surgery and then be done, but so much was happening that we were not prepared for.

By the time we left the hospital, it was six p.m. We hadn't even called the boys, who I knew were waiting to hear from us, nor had we eaten or drunk a thing all day except for a few sips of water. Our car was almost on the top floor of the garage, and I could see that Lee was spent, physically and emotionally, as we dragged ourselves up the five flights of stairs. I called Cryder from the car and he answered immediately.

"It's been a long day; we've been at Hopkins since eight this morning," I said, trying to figure out what to say.

But right away Cryder knew that something was wrong. As I spoke the tears just began. When I heard him say, "That's OK, Mom. I've just been worried," I lost all control and handed the phone to Lee. Amazingly, he explained everything to Cryder. Not once did his voice crack. *Be strong*, I urged myself.

Cryder just listened, and all I could think was that he had no one to hold and comfort him in that difficult moment. Being a very private person, I knew he would keep this to himself and not tell one of his five roommates. Thank God he had a girlfriend, who I knew would be there for him.

Just before Lee hung up I motioned for the phone. I mustered a few words of encouragement after Cryder admitted being "a little shocked."

"I know. A really big shock. But we have the best doctors, and Dad will fight this, don't you worry," I said, maybe as much for myself as for him. "He's a tough old guy, and I promise I will be fighting right alongside him. And he has you and Tim, too."

Lee was better rehearsed when he called Tim. I could tell there wasn't much talking on Tim's end, and that was unusual for Tim. He must have been stunned into silence. Again, I took the phone when Lee had finished. Tim was his usual comforting self, telling me it was going to be OK. He assured me Dad was tougher than he looked.

I so wanted both of our boys to be with us at that moment. It was a terrible way to tell them their father had cancer. It's not something that is easy to say at any time, but definitely harder over the phone.

I took what comfort I could in knowing that both boys had their girl-friends to confide in and comfort them when they needed it.

We were numb and exhausted by the time we got home. Still, we forced ourselves to eat some soup. As we reviewed everything we'd learned this awful day, we shared our thoughts and tried hard to be positive. It was what it was, and we would deal with it.

That night, when I lay in bed, trying to shut down my mind so I could get some sleep, I started reliving our meeting with Dr. Frassica. I finally understood the purpose of his question about my running and the will to do an Ironman. What I'd learned from all my endurance sports would be tested, because this was going to be a fight, not just for Lee, but for me as well. I think he wanted to know what I was made of, what I had inside me for this journey. He knew Lee would have to rely on my strength when his own faltered. Without a doubt, my running had affected all our lives, not only making me stronger, but my family, too, for experiencing the challenges and learning the lessons right alongside me.

Though this cancer sentence for Lee was overwhelming, I decided then and there that we would beat this thing, that I would be a positive influence on Lee and my whole family. This race would require everything I'd ever learned throughout my athletic career, and I was determined to get a handle on my fears and overcome what faced us. That was the reason for Dr. Frassica's question, I was sure of that.

14

And So It Begins—A New Race

The next morning when I woke I knew it was time to accept what was happening. First, I wrote a quick email to Tim to find out if he was planning to meet us in Chapel Hill for Cryder's lacrosse game that coming weekend. I was pretty sure that Tim was heading to Alaska for some back-country skiing, but was equally hoping he might abandon that trip in light of the situation with Lee. Tim was the greater risk-taker of our two sons, and having him off in the wilds of Alaska was adding to my level of anxiety, though I'd never tell Tim that.

The other email went to Cryder who was embarking on his final season of Division I UNC lacrosse, and Lee was afraid that he was going to ruin it for our son.

February 17, 2010
Morning, Cryder. I told Dad I'd send you an email because he's worried about you . . . he knows how similar you are to him, keeping things to yourself and worries you will shut down and stop caring about classes and lacrosse. Please stay focused on all that for him and make him proud. I know it is tough, but he loves you guys so much and knows how much we all love him and he will fight for us. Don't you worry. I am here anytime you want to talk. He is really looking forward to seeing you, so we'll have a good college weekend for him

and then move forward and attack this stupid tumor. I love you very much and am sending hugs and smiles your way.

xoxox

Mom

Writing to the boys gave me a boost. I read through the handful of emails awaiting me from friends wanting updates. I had a very moving email from Kitty, offering to do whatever she could to help and reminding me that I was strong, stubborn, and determined and I had to rely on those traits for Lee.

I got a little chuckle thinking about our childhood and my "redheaded temper" that sometimes Kitty feared when we had our sibling spats. I assured her I would rely on my fierce temperament and only let the tears flow when I was alone. I would respond to her email later and also send the group update that had to be written.

Lee seemed to have absorbed the news in his sleep and awoke with a new sense of determination. He was eager to make the calls to set up appointments for lung and pelvic scans and we began to take control of what we could.

I had a full day ahead but first checked my emails again hoping to hear back from the boys to know they were OK. I was so happy to read that Tim was coming to UNC to join us for the weekend, a perfect example of his compassionate side and sensitivity to other people's needs. Unfortunately, his long ago planned trip to Alaska meant he would leave the following Friday. As if he could read my mind, he assured me he'd be careful and said he, too, wished the timing were different.

Lee felt it was important to write an email to Cryder's lacrosse coach to let him know what was going on and keep an eye on Cryder. Coach Breschi had suffered a terrible hardship himself when he had lost his young son in an accident several years back. If things got tough, Coach Breschi would be a safety net for Cryder. Again, we were controlling what we could, and it felt empowering.

When Cryder wrote back, it brought tears to my eyes. He told me not to worry, that he would stay focused on his schoolwork and

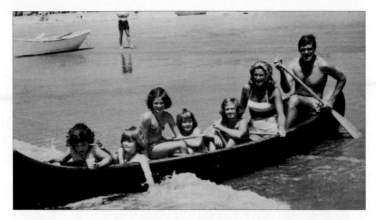

Summer of 1965 in Newport, Rhode Island with Mom, Dad, and my four sisters (I am the one in the middle, sitting up high).

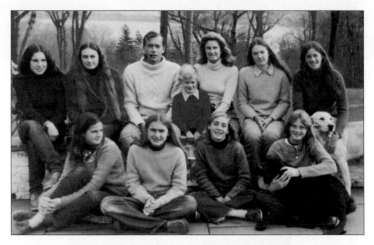

Fall of 1976 in Mill Neck, New York. Mom and Jack with their eight girls (five Cushing girls, three stepsisters) and Brewster.

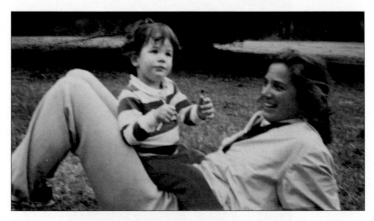

The last training run with Kitty before the 1985 Boston Marathon, being met by Tim in the field.

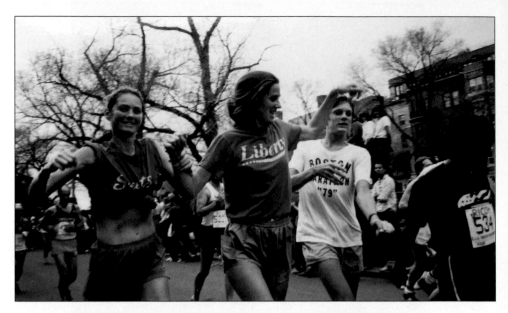

Nearing the finish line of the 1985 Boston Marathon with Kitty and Brewster.

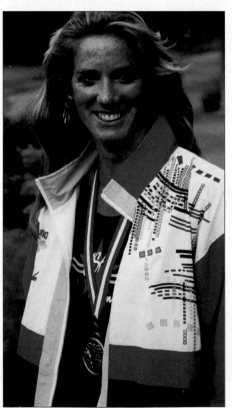

The 1993 Team USA uniform for World
Championships in Manchester, England.

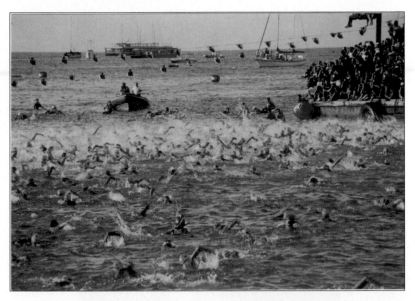

Swim start at the 1994 Ironman on the big island, Kailua Kona, Haiwaii.

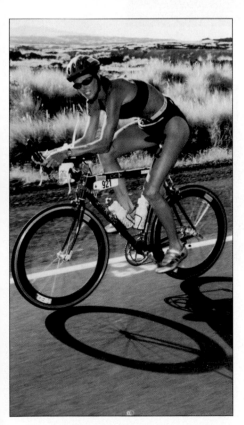

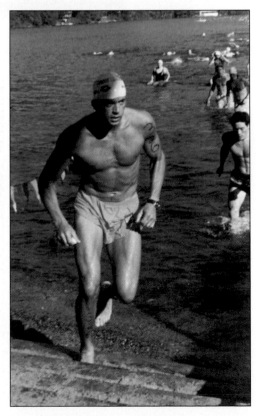

Riding down Queen K Highway
in the 1994 Ironman.

Lee exiting the swim at 1991 Fairlee,
Vermont, triathlon.

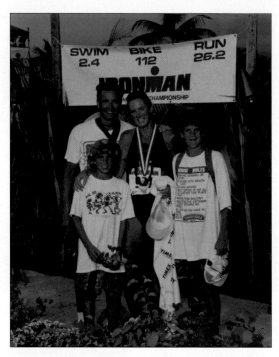

With Lee, Tim, and Cryder soon after I finished the
Hawaii Ironman.

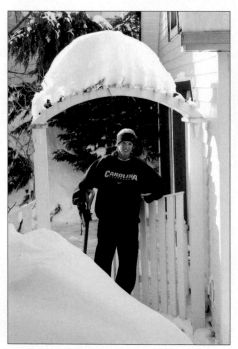

Februrary 2010. Diggin' out of continual
snowstorms at home in Maryland.

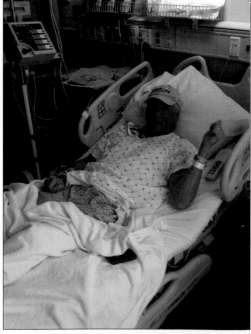

Lee beginning his chemotherapy treatments at
Johns Hopkins in February of 2010.

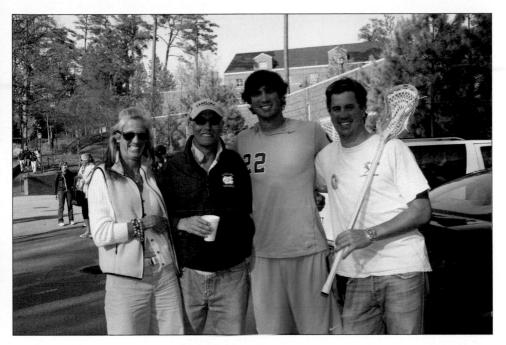

March 27, 2010, at a University of North Carolina tailgate with Lee, Tim, and Cryder

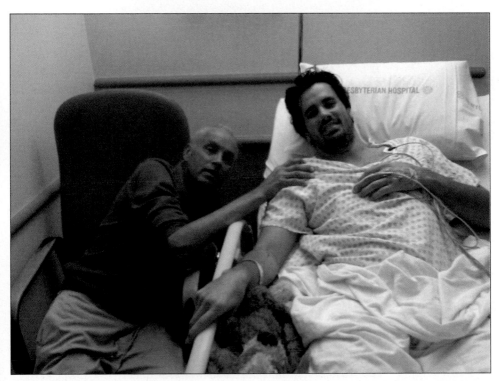

Lee and Tim at Hospital for Special Surgery, May 2010. It was the first reunion after Lee's surgery and Tim's accident.

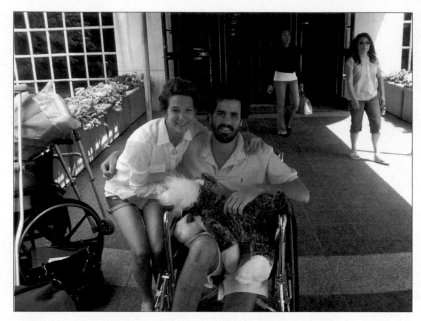

Memorial Day weekend with Gina, leaving hospital after Tim's almost four week stay.

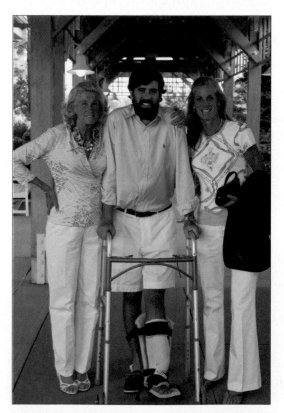

End of June 2010 . . . first night out! Tim with me and his grandmother Nina.

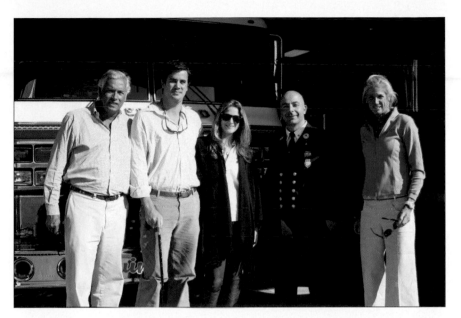

September 2010, meeting Lt. DiPietro with Lee, Tim, Gina, and myself.

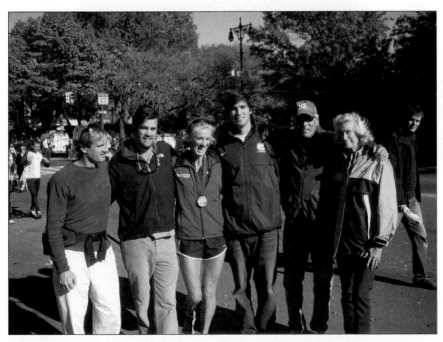

The finish at the New York City marathon in November of 2010, with Brewster, Tim, me, Cryder, Lee, and Mom.

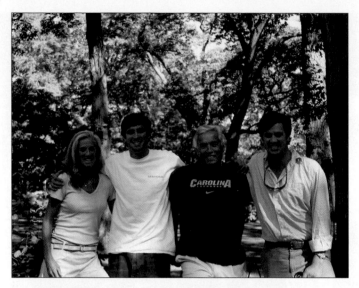

The healthy family!

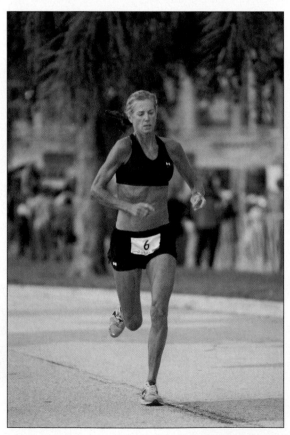

Winning the Palm Beach Marathon at age fifty!

lacrosse, and if anything, it would make him stay more focused. He wanted to make his father proud with a strong lacrosse season. I was so touched by both boys' concern for their father and me. They certainly had grown into mature, loving, and kind men. Cryder ended his email trying to make me laugh, as he often did, promising to go buy a Carolina Tar Heel blue wig for his dad to keep that shiny head warm when he lost his hair. Laughing was important too!

At the end of the day, chest and pelvic scans done, Lee was wiped out, and I finally found my way to the computer to write the group email that had been hanging over my head. Dated Wednesday, February 17, 2010, the email went out to a long list of friends and family and described, in some detail, all that had transpired in the hospital the previous day, as well as the chemo and radiation treatments Lee would undergo in preparation for the surgery to remove the tumor in his leg.

It amazed me how quickly the reply emails filled my inbox. The outpouring of love and support gave both of us a lift and I read each note to Lee, whose eyes brimmed with tears. The emotions were hard to hold back.

The following day, after we received the results of the chest and pelvic scans, I wrote another email to the full list.

February 18, 2010

Yesterday, Lee had chest and pelvic scans done. Before treatment could start, they had to ensure that no cancer cells had broken away from the tumor in his leg and traveled elsewhere. This was the third piece of the puzzle. Thank God, at this point the scans have come back clean. That was a huge relief. The radiologist was extremely informative and laid out the radiation procedure coupled with the chemo, and what we should expect as far as treatment and side effects. Lee had his game face on that said he was ready to go to battle!! As it looks now, he will report to Johns Hopkins at 8 a.m. on Monday to run some more tests and some more blood work. My poor pincushion!! He is due to get the port in his chest (for the chemo) at one and then hopefully he'll be admitted into the hospital to start the chemo treatments.

We are heading down to Chapel Hill tomorrow and really looking forward to a weekend "at college" (as Lee calls it!!) and a little time with Tim and Cryder. So please keep saying your prayers. I think it's working and someone is listening and afraid of the wrath of Nurse McNicey. Thanks again for all your thoughts and prayers.

The weekend in North Carolina was filled with good moments and also some harsh realities. With his boys at his side, Lee was in heaven; and of course a little dose of love was great for me as well. I had the extra duty, though, of telling everyone who hadn't known about Lee's illness and what he faced, which had to be done but was stressful. Again, people were incredibly supportive and wanted to know what they could do.

On the negative side, Lee was easily tired over the course of the weekend and snapped at me more than once. Finally, I decided it was time for a little chat. I told him I was devastated for him and didn't know how I could make it better. I was more than aware of the fatigue, the frustration, and his fears, and I would do everything I could, but he had to fight with me, not against me. I could not take the punishment for his illness. It was not my fault.

I knew I was being a bit harsh, but he needed a pep talk. I didn't want him to waste energy feeling sorry for himself or being angry. He needed to use all his inner resources to fight this thing, and I would be right beside him every step. It was a tough moment, but as always he appreciated my honesty and understood my position. It is so hard to be the healthy one and watch your spouse have to accept what has happened. A part of me was dying inside for him, but I couldn't let him know that.

In preparation for the first of his three hospital stays for the week-long chemo treatments, we tried to figure out what he should bring. Did he need pajamas? Would he feel well enough to read a book? In the end, he packed his flannel PJs, and I threw in a book, just in case.

Dinner that night was quiet; both of us struggling with our thoughts. We stared at the TV for a while, but eventually we talked about what was to come. In a strange way, he was excited to get started, and I realized I felt the same way. The cancer was there, still growing, but now we were going after it.

The next morning, as we drove down to Hopkins, we were both feeling overwhelmed with fear and anticipation about getting the process started. What would Lee's reaction to the drugs be? I had barely slept, saying prayers every time I rolled over. Lee tossed and turned, too. He was sweating through T-shirts, as he had been doing for weeks. But, of course, there was much on his mind. He had seen his father battle cancer and watched as it slowly beat him down, then take his life.

I had been married to Lee when his father died and knew how horrible and difficult it had been. On our drive to the hospital that morning, though, neither of us said of any of this. I'm sure Lee was fearful, but hoped he didn't have those images in his head. Anyway, this was D-day, the day we were beginning the fight. It was a new race.

Johns Hopkins Hospital is like a small city. Just finding your way around can be a challenge. His first appointment was with radiology in the basement of the Weinberg Building. It was early and we were the first to arrive. I couldn't go in with him, but afterward Lee said the radiation simulation was a bit uncomfortable. They had to make a "form" for him to lie on so the radiation could be delivered to the same spot each time. He would also be "tattooed" to direct the radiation to the correct spots each time (for fifteen minutes on each of five days in a row, then the weekend off, then five days in a row again, following each round of chemo). The best way to get to the right position was for him to lie on his back with his knees bent and falling open to either side. Not a comfortable—or modest—position, for sure. I guess it's like having a baby: after a while, you really don't care who's seeing what as long as the outcome is favorable!

It turned out to be another long day of going from one appointment to the next. Lee seemed in a trance and let me lead him to each office without question.

His last appointment at two in the afternoon was for a surgical procedure to insert a Hickman line for the chemotherapy treatments. This was in an older, rather rundown section of Hopkins, not the clean, fancy cancer wing. The waiting room was cramped, and the metal and vinyl chairs were worn and uncomfortable. The TV was on way too loud, and then a large woman arrived with a greasy brown bag smelling of something awful. She planted herself right across from me with her knees almost touching mine, then started eating whatever was inside that bag. Moments later, a young boy in a wheelchair arrived. He was hooked up to all kinds of lines and monitors but appeared to be used to this routine. I had to keep myself from stealing glances at him; it was so sad to see a child like that.

I was very happy when they finally called my name around four o'clock to tell me Lee was being taken from surgery to his room in the cancer center. I could go with them, which was good! I had enough of sitting in that depressing waiting room.

It was a strange feeling, walking alongside Lee in his hospital bed as he was being wheeled by a tiny black woman chatting up a storm. Lee was still pretty out of it, not listening to her, but she was hysterical and entertaining. It was a relief to laugh a little. As the three of us made our way down the main hallway of the hospital, past the cafeteria and to the elevator up to the cancer center, I could see some people stealing glances at us, but most were oblivious. In weeks to come, this would feel normal and I too would feel familiar here.

On Lee's floor everything was clean and sterile. A nurse's station was situated in the center of sixteen rooms, each one with windows. Lee's had a view of downtown Baltimore and this would be his home for the week. Inside the doorway of each room was a sink, with cabinets above and below, and also liquid sanitizer hand pumps (they were everywhere in the hospital) and a pile of surgical masks. Every time I entered his room, I had to clean my hands and wear a surgical mask. Everything had to be kept sterile.

While the nurses were settling Lee into his room, I waited in the corner, trying to stay out of the way. When they left, I unpacked Lee's things. He had brought a photo of the boys and me that he wanted on his bedside. Needless to say, I was touched! I called to get his TV turned on and then got him all tucked in. I stayed with him until around six thirty when he finally threw me out. His first chemo treatment was scheduled for that night, but he was in good hands. As much as I hated to leave him, it was time to go. Once again, I'd had little to eat and discovered I was light-headed from lack of food.

When I got home around seven o'clock, though, I went straight to the basement to ride my stationary bike. I had all this pent-up energy and needed to get the hospital out of my system. My legs were spinning on the bike as fast as they could go. I was surely riding away from something. After about forty minutes, I'd worked up a good sweat. A hot shower completed the cleansing process. But I couldn't stop thinking about the drugs that were about to enter Lee's body. I turned on the TV to distract my thoughts and to help me fall asleep. It was another tough night of tossing and turning, continually waking, wondering how Lee was doing.

Tuesday morning I woke very early and finally decided to get up and check my emails. Family and friends were very concerned and sending good wishes. Though it was difficult to answer them all, it meant so much to hear from so many people. The constant flow of emails kept me in touch with the real world of friends and family, and reminded me that we were important to them, too. I preferred emailing over speaking on the phone as I found it so much easier to share my feelings in writing, and I also started to realize that these emails were becoming a release for me. By writing down all the things that were happening and then pushing "Send," I was getting rid of the burden in some way. It was odd, but I felt better after I wrote, and I loved getting all the replies. It felt as if we were sharing our burden, and Lee loved hearing me read them to him.

The emails were a terrific form of support, but I also needed my morning run to face the day. I waited for the first sign of light to throw on my shoes and race out the door. Adrenaline was keeping my energy level high and allowing me my therapy on the roads. What would I have done without my running? It kept me feeling alive and my blood pumping. After the run, I couldn't wait to get to the hospital to see how Lee was doing.

15

Fast Track/Slow Track

My mother had offered several times to come to Baltimore when Lee started chemo, and each time I'd declined, knowing Lee was scared and would need to conserve his energy. But Lee and Mom were also extremely close, so, in Mom's typical fashion, "no" was not an answer she accepted. She was arriving Tuesday afternoon, Lee's second day of treatment, to bring him a Kindle. That was the excuse she'd offered for her visit, not only to deliver it but also to show him how to use it.

But I suspected there was another reason my mother planned to come. About thirteen years ago, she too had suffered from cancer. Despite being only fifty-six, healthy, athletic, and vibrant, like many women her age, she'd been diagnosed with breast cancer. She received a double mastectomy and weeks of radiation. I was at her side while she went through this (we lived next door at the time) and every day I reminded her she was still beautiful. Six years later, in 1996, she stood beside me after I'd finished my second Hawaii Ironman and confessed to feeling miserable because of the side effects of tamoxifen, which she'd been taking for five years to replace her estrogen. It made her feel fat and bloated, she said. I had to laugh because Mom had never been fat except the six times she was pregnant.

I stepped in. "Well, let's fix that. I'll start you on a walking program to lose that weight."

"Walking?" she said in a horrified tone. "Walk? I want to run!" Of course she did. She was an avid tennis player and extremely competitive in everything she did. I suppose I had to have gotten those competitive genes from somewhere.

"All right then," I said with a laugh. "Run it is."

About a year later, in October 1997, we entered the Race for the Cure in Baltimore, a 5k race devoted to raising money for breast cancer. Mom was sixty-three years old. On the morning of the race she was a bundle of nerves and began to doubt herself. I recognized those pre-race jitters but knew they would give her a burst of adrenaline and help her make it to the finish line. We reviewed the plan; I reminded her to start slow and stick to her pace, not to get caught up in someone else's race. She agreed, but she also made a deal with me.

"Okay," she said, "I'll finish, but only if you win!"

I'd come in second (female) the previous year, but this was a very competitive race with thousands of runners, so I had my work cut out for me. The streets of downtown Baltimore were crowded with spectators, and to my surprise the race had arranged for six Hell's Angels-type motorcyclists to escort the lead woman to the finish. Well, as it turned out, that woman was me.

After crossing the finish line, I immediately turned back, jogging along the course to find Mom and escort her to the end. When I spotted her at the two-mile mark as planned, she immediately asked if I'd won. "Yes," I beamed, and now she knew she had to finish. Her determination drew her to the finish as I ran alongside encouraging her every step. The look on her face when she made her goal was priceless—a huge smile that couldn't be contained.

Now, I sensed, she was here for both Lee and me as proof of survival. And interestingly, Lee was the same age as Mom when she'd been diagnosed and had her own battle with cancer! So not only had she gone on to run in that race and other 5k's almost every year, but she'd also been a cancer survivor for twenty years. What a perfect message to deliver to Lee! And to me.

Since she wasn't arriving until late afternoon, I snuck into the hospital a little before visiting hours began at ten. I had something special to bring Lee for breakfast: his favorite coffee cake made by a good friend. At least I knew that this would make him happy to see me!

I spent the morning sitting by his bed, occasionally staring outside at the Baltimore skyline. When he dozed, I picked up my book and waited for him to wake up again. Sometimes, I left the room for a few minutes to remove the surgical mask visitors were required to wear. It was a suffocating feeling to have that mask over my nose and mouth, and the elastic bands that went behind the ears also began to irritate my skin. I don't know how the nurses kept them on as long as they did—perhaps they had formed calluses behind their ears!

One of the things the nurses encouraged the patients to do was to get some exercise. Now that was right up my alley! But it was challenging as Lee had four different bags of fluid hanging on his IV pole. (By the way, when the nurses changed the chemo bag, they had to be dressed in HAZMAT attire because the chemicals were so very toxic. A bit scary knowing that this stuff was flowing through Lee's veins.) They told us we could go for walks around the Weinberg Wing. However, we could not leave the square hallway that surrounded the nurse's station. I decided we should give our IV pole a name—after all, it would be accompanying Lee wherever he went—and so we dubbed him Stanley. That's the name that popped into my head for no apparent reason, but it did and it stuck!

Late that morning, we set out for a walk. I grabbed hold of Stanley and told him to move along because he was holding us up. Happily, I could take my mask off, but, unfortunately out here Lee had to wear one. As we walked past all the rooms, we noticed dates on the patient's doors and realized some had already been in the hospital for weeks. Suddenly, we felt lucky. As we rounded the last corner, I noticed a chart on the wall. It listed all the patients' names and the number of laps they had done in a day. Oh, boy! Competition! I studied the chart to find the person with the most laps and excitedly told Lee I was sure he could beat that number. He couldn't help but laugh.

When Mom arrived, I realized just how much I needed her. Just seeing her smile and feeling the warmth and love from her hug renewed my strength. She arrived with my favorite oatmeal cookies, carrot bread, and other things to fatten me up. And of course she brought Lee's favorite gingersnaps.

Lee was all smiles when we walked into his hospital room, and Mom was amazed by how great he looked. We laughed and joked, especially when she tried to explain how to use the Kindle. Jack had given her instructions, which she had scribbled on a small piece of paper, but her technology skills were limited, to say the least. It made us laugh when not even she could decipher her notes.

Sadly, she had to leave first thing in the morning. Ironically, Jack was having a surgery that afternoon. It was a simple outpatient procedure, but she wanted to be there for him. We had a cup of coffee in our kitchen before she left, trying to extend our little time together for a few more minutes. My eyes filled with tears as she hugged me goodbye. As she turned out of our driveway in Ruxton, I felt as though my other half was leaving and the strength and comfort she'd brought was leaving with her. Still, she'd accomplished her mission, giving us both love and the courage to see things through.

February 2, 2010

Morning, everyone. Quick update. Lee had to have a blood transfusion because his red cell count was less than half of what it should be and he was extremely anemic. I spent most of the day with him yesterday and so far . . . no bad side effects. He is holding his breath, hoping he will be able to handle the chemo. A group of doctors and interns (Hopkins is a teaching hospital) came in for rounds when I was there. (Don't worry, Nurse McNicey spotted them at the door before they came in and made sure our boy was covered up and hair all spoofed up!!) All in all, it was a good day. I think he feels he has taken a huge step forward in fighting this monster and is in good spirits. Again, we are so appreciative of all the calls and emails and notes and food. We feel so loved. Thank you!

 xoxox

All went well until Thursday morning, Lee's third day of chemo, when he developed a serious case of the hiccups. Before I left for the hospital he called me and said he was also starting to feel "heavy," which worried me. I fully expected to find out he'd been throwing up all night. When I turned the doorknob to his room, I mustered all my positive thoughts and put on my best smile.

"Morning," I said in my most enthusiastic voice. Only he wasn't looking so good.

The hiccups had worn him out. I began trying every crazy remedy I could think of, from scaring him to making him drink water with his chin tilted towards his chest while sipping from the back of the glass. Not surprisingly, nothing worked.

Finally, that night he asked the nurses if there was anything they could suggest. For chronic hiccups, they said they used a drug called Thorazine, which they gave him at 10:30 p.m. Within a short amount of time, he was hallucinating! Apparently it's a drug used to treat mentally ill patients. When I called him the next morning before leaving for the hospital, he was still feeling totally out of it. He said he'd been dreaming about the book *Shutter Island* all night and had found himself wandering the dark halls with old, dead patients from Hopkins.

By the time I arrived, he was still feeling hung over and slept most of the day. But besides feeling really tired he was doing great. Still, no nausea. I planned to leave early to attend Cryder's game in Annapolis against Navy. When it was time to leave, I had Lee all set up with his laptop nearby, so he could follow the game. He was a huge fan and had thrown a few of his luckiest garments in his suitcase—his Vineyard Vines Tar Heel boxers and his #22 UNC lacrosse hat (Cryder's number). I left him all dressed and ready for the game.

That night, as was predicted, it was freezing cold with winds gusting up to 45 mph. The boys played great, but in the last quarter, because they had built up a good lead, most of the starting players were pulled and had to stand on the sidelines in their sweaty wet clothes. I could see Cryder's whole body shaking. After the game ended, the teams shook hands as fast as they could and made a dash for the locker rooms. I had to see Cryder before the bus took him back to UNC to give him a congratulatory hug and to make sure he was hanging tough.

The wind was blowing so hard that I could hardly make it to my car. I drove around to the back of the stadium where it was really dark, but I finally found the lot where the bus was parked and started calling Cryder's cell phone. He answered right away and told me to run toward the bus so he could see me. With my cell phone to my ear, I was yelling over the roar of the wind, "I'm over here—do you see me?"

At six feet four inches, Cryder was easy to see as he dashed across the parking lot. We ran and met each other with a big hug. "I'm so proud of you guys. You played great!"

"Thanks, Mom. You OK?"

"Yeah, I'm OK. You OK?"

"Yup, thanks for coming. Gotta go! Bus is leaving."

"Love you," I yelled.

"Love you, too!"

That was it; just a minute together and a hug, but I wouldn't have missed it for the world.

On Friday morning, I woke up feeling a bit apprehensive. Tim was leaving for Alaska with a group of his guy pals. It was his dream trip with a week of backcountry skiing and a day of heli-skiing, but from my perspective too many things could happen on such adventure trips, and Tim always seemed to attract the outcomes you don't want! A thrill-seeker, my brother called him, an adrenaline junkie.

It was true, Tim was my adventure child *and* an amazing skier. That was his passion. But he didn't just ski down a hill. He loved to jump off cliffs and launch himself straight down the mountain. He had threatened for years to do a back flip on skis. I would always say, "Tim, please don't do that. You could land on your head and end up in a wheelchair for the rest of your life. Is it really worth it? Think about what could happen." And often something did happen.

One spring when he was in college—and no longer the skinny 150-pound teen who would taunt me with his intent to try back flips—Tim went out west to ski. He was not only bigger but probably a wee bit out of shape. One afternoon, I got a phone call.

"Hey, Mom, it's me!" He was breathless and obviously very excited about something. "I just landed my first back flip!"

I was silent for a minute. Stunned, in fact.

"But don't worry, Mom. As I was launching myself down the hill, I did hear your voice in my head saying, 'Tim, don't do this!'"

It took me a second to respond. "Well, that's great, but that was not the time you should have been hearing my voice say 'Don't do this.' It was *before* you launched yourself that you should have listened to me. Holy moly, Tim, you are a dope!"

We both laughed. His life was full of stories like that, some that ended happily, but also ones that ended with injuries.

Now that he was an adult, I often wanted to tell Tim not to be such a risk-taker, though I also knew the importance of him following his dreams. As he often reminded me with a laugh, no one told you that you couldn't fly off to Hawaii and take the risks you did when competing in an Ironman. And, of course, he was right. Now all I wanted was for him to go and then come home safely.

Though afraid for Tim, I was also excited, because today I would spring Lee from Hopkins and bring him home. I was so hoping he'd made it through the night without too many ill effects. We still didn't know what to expect from that poison running through his veins.

When I arrived in his room, he was anxiously waiting for me. He was ready to go! I received a lengthy list of instructions. I was amazed at how much had to be done. I asked the nurse what patients did if they didn't have a spouse or someone to care for them. She shrugged and said they had to find someone. Being alone and sick—what a terrible thought.

It seemed like forever before we got the paper work done and all the prescriptions filled. Finally, Lee was released. I grabbed all his bags and we headed for the elevator. When the doors closed, he leaned over and gave me a teary-eyed kiss.

"One session down, two to go," I said and gave him a big hug. Then he released another hiccup!

16

Swan Song—Ironman Canada 2000

Lee and I had been a team for a long time. In all my years of racing and training, Lee was always there as a sounding board, a therapist, a trainer, a coach, and, most importantly, my watchful protector. He worried when I disappeared for long training runs, watching the clock to make sure I came home when expected. He knew my pace, my running form, my body language. If I showed any signs of injury, he noticed. I couldn't hide anything from him! Plus, I was a terrible patient when I did get hurt. Taking time off to repair an injury is something most runners are not good at, which is what I discovered about myself in August, when I arrived in Penticton, British Columbia, to race in the Ironman Canada 2000.

At this point in my racing career I'd finished a total of 146 triathlons and duathlons over a period of twelve years. Ironman Canada would be my sixth Ironman (the first had been six years earlier), and I vowed it would be my swan song. Earlier in the year, when I'd mapped out my racing season, I asked Lee for one more favor, to join me on one more Ironman and then I'd hang up my hat. In fact, I said I would retire from all triathlon racing, but hopefully go out with a bang.

This was not an easy decision, but one I had to make for my family's sake. The past six years of racing as a professional triathlete had had its wearing effect, not only on me, emotionally and physically (the pressure to win was high), but also on my family. By 2000, our sons were thirteen and seventeen, and they'd tired of having to plan vacations and weekend activities around my racing schedule. When we went to Florida, for example, our days still had to include my training while they sat and waited for me to return. My emotional ups and downs related to racing affected them too. And, Lee, well, he mostly got frustrated and felt neglected when I was exhausted and would fall asleep on the sofa at nine!

I'd had a good run and we'd all made sacrifices, each in our own ways. But triathlons, especially Ironmans, could be all consuming, so I knew it was time to quit.

Arriving in Penticton, I wasn't so confident, knowing I'd had a serious setback in the spring. I had been in great shape, racing well and racing often through the late winter and early spring months. On the last weekend of April I ran a very competitive 10k (I came in first in the Masters) in Washington, DC, and in my typical fashion I hurried off the podium so I could participate in family events in the afternoon. I sped home, ran upstairs, and jumped in the shower. In my continued rush, I stepped out of the shower onto the tile floor where my foot slid forward as if I were stepping on an ice rink, and then I was thrown backwards as I caught myself on the counter. I felt the shooting pain immediately run from my groin down the front of my right leg.

Of course I ignored the pain and tried to run the next day, and the next, but the pain was too great and I succumbed to seeing a doctor who delivered the dreaded news. I'd torn something deep in my groin and there would be no running for at least eight or more weeks. This was a real blow and something I was not accustomed to dealing with as an athlete. To this point in my career, I had been very lucky, having dealt with only slight injuries here and there, certainly nothing major like this.

I was furious with myself, but I did what I could to stay in shape, with lots of "water running," increased mileage on the bike, and regular physical therapy. After nine weeks, I was approved to run again. I tested myself in a sprint triathlon in Connecticut on July 22, coming in second among the women, and then again in Wilkes-Barre,

Pennsylvania, early in August in a very competitive triathlon where I finished fourth among the professional females. That confirmed I was back in racing form. After Wilkes-Barre, though, I still worried that I was significantly behind the fitness level I should be in approaching an Ironman. Deep down, I knew it would be a huge challenge and I just hoped and prayed my body could withstand the grueling race.

Lee had come to cheer me on once again and celebrate my last triathlon together. He knew well my concerns and tried to brush them off as I did, not wanting to allow any doubt to creep in before the race.

Early on race morning, as the sun began to rise, I stood in line for the ritual of body marking, where volunteers use black magic markers to write your race number on your arm, the front of your thighs, and on your calves. Then I continued on to where my bike was racked in the transition area.

As always, my nerves had me on edge and so I tried to calm myself, following my well-honed routine: check my bike, make sure the tires are blown up to the proper pounds per square inch, pour Accelerade into the plastic bottle mounted between my handlebars, peel off chunks of power bars and stick them to my bike frame for easy access, and finally place my helmet, glasses, and bike shoes in ready position for a quick transition after the swim.

I checked and double-checked all my equipment, grabbed my wetsuit, and went to look for Lee on the other side of the fenced-in transition area where only the athletes were allowed to enter. He was watching for me, waved me over, and gave me his usual pre-race pep talk.

"Go get 'em, champ. You're going to be great!"

"Thanks," I said with a relieved yet nervous exhale. I leaned over the fence to give him a hug and kiss and one last squeeze for reassurance before I turned towards the lake with my wetsuit in hand. The swim has always been the worst part for me, knowing I'll get bumped, dunked, and swum over while trying to find my space for the 2.4-mile swim among the other 1,500 athletes.

But this morning was a little different and bittersweet knowing it was my last time. I looked over the lake and at the slight mist rising from the water and thought to myself: *I've had a good ride*. But this wasn't the time to be nostalgic—I had a job to do. Then came my pep talk to myself: *Hang tough, find your ribbon of space, and swim strong.*

I positioned myself near a group of women that I could pace myself with on the swim. Once the gun goes off, it's bedlam and impossible to find the people you want to swim with. I always preferred being with the women as the men tended to be much more aggressive.

"*Bang*," and we were off. I dolphined into the lake, holding my ground as my nerves settled in. I thought I was doing okay, but when I came out of the lake, eyeing the timing clock near the swim exit, it read sixty-five minutes, a good five to seven minutes slower than I was hoping for. *Damn it*, I thought, *move it Lee!*

I'm pretty quick with my transitions and soon was on my bike and heading out of town, though still feeling a little chilled and dizzy from the water. With my heart pounding hard, I told myself to relax and get into a rhythm for the long haul on the bike.

But I couldn't seem to get into a smooth pedal stroke. I geared down to an easier gear instead of fighting the harder gears. Still, I was getting easily passed, and fatigue was coming too early in the race. About forty miles into the biking, I couldn't seem to get into a comfortable position and a sharp pain settled into my lower right back. I tried to reposition myself, but the pain continued. It took a little more time before I realized why my back was seemingly in spasm. I'd been feeling as if I was tilting to one side but had ignored this. In fact, the stem to one of my elbow cups on my carbon fiber aerobars had snapped, causing me to ride in a slightly crooked position instead of the aerodynamic position that allows the bicyclist to achieve faster speeds and better efficiency.

Well, this was definitely going to be a problem, especially since I still had seventy miles to ride. Plus, now I had to resort to sitting upright and crouching down as much as possible. Not a very comfortable position. And that wasn't the only issue. For some reason, I had a constant urge to pee. Over the years, I had learned to relieve myself while riding—I know, not something I should be proud of, but this is part of our sport that the cameras hopefully don't share with the spectators! In any case, I was getting increasingly concerned that I wasn't staying hydrated and all the fluid I was drinking was going right through me. *Keep riding, just keep riding*, I told myself. I also kept checking my watch and discovered that I was losing time, and confidence.

The last thirty miles, we had to ride dead into the wind. Without the ability to get down on my aerobars, the wind was catching me right in the chest and it seemed like I was fighting a losing battle. As frustrated as I was, I did what I could to keep my head down and fight through this wind tunnel. Finally at the top of the last long steep hill that led into town, I thought, *Phew, almost there, one more downhill.* But then, as I started down the hill, hitting about twenty miles an hour, my front wheel started to wobble uncontrollably. *Oh my God, please don't let me crash*, I thought, as I pumped the brakes the way you do on an icy road, until the bike stopped. I got off, checked the wheel lock and alignment of the wheel, then checked everything else I knew to check, and with fear running through me, I got back into the saddle and slowly resumed rolling down the hill, silently praying my wheel would remain stable.

At last, I made it back to the dismount area and immediately heard the concern in Lee's voice as he spotted me. "Are you okay," he yelled as I ran past him into the transition area and out again. "Hang in there, babe," he yelled again, and my heart began pounding. The adrenaline rush sent me out on the 26.2-mile run. I was now at least thirty minutes behind where I wanted to be and I was worried, especially since I wasn't in my usual running shape. My legs were stiff, as expected, and was I telling myself to feel the rhythm, spring from step to step, when Lee rode up behind me on the bike.

"You okay? What happened?"

I briefly explained the trouble on the bike, but didn't want to waste energy talking and, of course, he wasn't allowed to ride alongside me for more than a few seconds at a time. I assured him I was fine and ran off down the road.

It was a long, hard run, but I managed to make up some time on the other women and did manage to run myself from about thirtieth place (after the bike ride), back into ninth place (overall female). Needless to say, I was truly disappointed that I didn't have a stellar race to commemorate a great career. I wanted to pay tribute to this sport that had taught me so much about myself and, at times, allowed me to be a star. But it was fitting that my last race had taught me another important lesson about the strength and perseverance I had called on so many times. It was one of the reasons I loved this sport so much, it allowed me to test myself and prove to myself over and over that I *can* do what I set out to do.

Driving away from Penticton two days later, I stared out the window as our car climbed away from town, away from the lake, and up the same hill I almost crashed on. I was silent and Lee let me be. My heart felt heavy. I was leaving a life that had been so much a part of me. So many memories ran through my mind that it was like watching an old movie reel of races and friends and the many places we had been.

Now Lee would have to tap into his own reservoir of strength and perseverance, and I would have to put up with his moody temperament, as he'd once put up with mine when I'd taken time off to recover from an injury. I just hoped I could be as patient with his healing process as he had been with mine.

17

A New Routine

The first weekend after Lee's chemo involved a lot of trial and error, especially surrounding food. I felt like something of an expert since I'd dealt with nutritional issues—balancing carbohydrates, protein, and fat—for my training and racing. The problem for Lee was that he didn't have much of an appetite; the chemo had destroyed that along with his taste buds. Since nothing really tasted good, he had already lost about fifteen pounds, which worried me since this was only the beginning of his treatments. I did try to offer him some of his favorite meals, and he did his best to choke them down.

Boost, a drink that increases protein and calories, became his friend and was recommended by Dr. Deborah Frassica, Lee's radiologist and Dr. Frank Frassica's wife. She explained that other patients found liquids easier to stomach than solid foods. That made sense to me because when I raced I couldn't stomach solid food the morning of the race or during a race, and not for several hours after.

But these were only a few of the things that challenged us and changed our lives dramatically.

Though Lee was told that he could do whatever he felt capable of doing and that it was important he try to keep up his strength with exercise, sitting around would occupy much of our time. Obviously, for a while we would no longer maintain our golf routine (tennis had already gone by the wayside), nor could he continue biking. The location of the sarcoma limited his ability to sit on a bicycle. He could also continue going to work if he felt up to it, which he did but only for a few hours at a time. It was important to make life as normal for Lee as possible, and when we succeeded he always felt better.

However, an unfortunate by-product that plagued Lee during the first round of chemo was the "chemo hiccups," which affect about thirty percent of chemo patients, mostly men. But even after the chemo they continued with a vengeance. I never thought anyone could die from hiccupping, but it suddenly seemed like Lee might be the first victim. And surprisingly, the doctors had little advice on how to cure them.

For a time, we were flooded with friends' suggestions of how to rid him of the hiccups, but nothing seemed to work. I spent hours on the Internet looking for a cure. Several of the sites recommended an antispasmodic or a muscle relaxer. Apparently the anti-nausea medication is what causes the upper respiratory spasms to occur. The question occurring to us: which was the lesser of the two evils? We were hoping, as the effects of the chemo filtered through his body, that the hiccups would subside.

The scariest part was the way the hiccups built and built and then suddenly Lee's throat would close and he'd begin gasping for air, almost as if the wind had just gotten knocked out of him. It was especially scary at night. I lay awake and listened to the pattern of his hiccups and anticipate the gasping. Then I'd grab him by the arm, pull him up so he could breathe and slap him hard on the back to break the spasm. For some reason, the hiccups seemed to stop after that gasp and he'd fall back to sleep. I, however, could not! I lay there watching his chest to see if it was moving and holding my hand under his nose to make sure he was still breathing.

But I had many other duties, including having to give Lee a shot every fourteen days. *Wow, another step for McNicey*, I wrote to my friends. Friday was time to change Lee's bandage around his port, so I carefully placed all my equipment on the table next to him as he lay on the sofa. I put everything in sequential order to make sure I did every step correctly. I was getting to be a pro. Even Lee was impressed with my skillful nursing!

The following week Lee went to the office for a few hours and was happy to put his brain back to work and to see his colleagues. The doctors said he could do whatever he felt up to, though no vacuuming or ironing (because of the port in his chest), as if my husband regularly helped with such chores! At one point, Lee compared his radiation treatments to the movie *Independence Day*—the radiation rays were destroying the alien craft!

Whenever I could fit in my daily run, I did. It was like being in my own church doing my own praying. And I appreciated immensely the support of our family and friends—their emails, prayers, and concern.

But I was also learning to troubleshoot Lee's problems. It was something I learned early in my triathlon career after Lee hired my first coach, Hank Lang. I recall driving up to Vermont to meet with him. We went through all sorts of testing, videotaping me while biking, swimming, and running. Then we were about to embark on a thirty mile bike ride together. By this time, I felt totally exhausted and overwhelmed and nervous. I got my bike off the back of the car and joined him in the driveway. He was going to check the fitting on the bike, the gears, and so on. The first thing he asked me was, "Where's your spare tire and pump? What are you planning to do if we get a flat on our ride? Take my spare tube? I don't think so. It'll be a long walk home for you!"

Well, that took the feet out from under me. He said you have to learn to troubleshoot in this sport. There will always be times when something happens, whether during training or in a race, and you might be out in the middle of nowhere with no one to help you but yourself. So you have to assess the situation and start thinking of solutions. Be prepared for what might happen and have a plan to fix it. Because giving up is not what this is all about.

That lesson really stuck with me and I began to apply that mentality to all of life. Now, more than ever, I was faced with assessing Lee's situation and coming up with solutions.

For example, that weekend we woke up to a chilly and windy UNC game day. In the past, on cold days like this one, Lee would wrap his arms around me to keep me warm. But now our roles had reversed. He got cold easily, and so I had brought hats, gloves, warm jackets, and blankets to keep him warm. Despite my efforts, he still shivered.

An hour after the game, the boys were back in the bus heading home to North Carolina while we sped off in the opposite direction to meet with some of the parents in a local bar to celebrate our win. Lee thought we should join them; I knew he was insisting on my behalf, but I was looking forward to spending some time with friends and seeing Lee laugh. And laugh he did. Then a miracle happened. Lee's hiccups, after ten days of non-stop hiccupping, were about to meet their match.

A friend and one of the UNC parents, Paul Delaney, is a chiropractor. He explained how the phrenic nerve runs along the esophagus. (Of course, as Lee's nurse, I had already read up on and *knew* that!) The phrenic nerve controls the diaphragm, which in turn can cause the hiccups. With his fingertips, Paul put pressure on the phrenic nerve running down his neck. The nerve relaxed and poof: hiccups gone! Paul showed me how to do this in case the hiccups returned, which they probably would once the chemo started again. I did practice this method with Paul watching. I wrapped my fingers around Lee's neck and got ready to squeeze when another UNC dad looked over and said, "Oh my God! McNicey is trying to strangle him!" Hmmmm, I thought, possibly another cure!

Finally, on Sunday, Tim was due to fly out of Alaska via Chicago. I hadn't spoken to him since he left. A year earlier, Tim had gone out west to ski and had fallen and shattered his collarbone. Now, when the phone rang that afternoon showing Tim's caller ID, my heart raced as I answered. He was fine. Thank goodness, because I don't think I could have handled any more problems just then. On and off, I was also worrying about some additional blood tests they'd decided to run because of inconclusive results they'd found in Lee's bone marrow. In any case, that night I rested easier and was very grateful that Tim had returned safely, but it would not be the last time that Tim's "live life and follow your dreams" motto was put to the test.

For me, life was getting crazy as I juggled taking care of Lee, managing the house, paying bills, answering endless emails, organizing traveling to Cryder's lacrosse games, arranging hotels and dinners, and, at the bottom of the list, taking care of myself. I needed more energy than I could imagine, and yet somehow I was rising to the occasion. Another thing on the horizon was Cryder's team dinner that we'd offered to host, and which I had volunteered to be in charge of. Though other mothers had offered to take my place and I knew that the timing was off, I decided to honor that commitment. I wanted normalcy, too, and in a strange way this provided it!

It was the second week of radiation, and Lee seemed to be bouncing back from the chemo. He was handling the fatigue well. He wanted to take control of his body so he started exercising to show who was boss. Good boy! I offered to go on walks with him. "We'll start slowly," I promised. We went at his pace. He grew breathless easily, but he was determined. Amazing how quickly this disease had weakened him. A man who used to be a triathlete, golfer, tennis player, skier, you name it, could now only walk for about twenty minutes, if that. But I was proud of him. He was not giving up!

A few days later though he began losing his wonderful curly hair and he felt momentarily demoralized and off balance. So did I when I noticed strands of hair all over his pillow.

In one of my emails I wrote:

> I didn't want to say anything . . . but the inevitable is happening. He went to brush his hair and called me into the bathroom, alarmed at all the hair in the brush. He left for work with his cap on his head . . . looking a bit down. He came home before his radiation and sat on the porch with me, enjoying a beautiful spring day. He turned to me with tears in his eyes and said he was really upset about his hair starting to come out. My heart sank for him, but I assured

him he has a beautiful head and still has the same handsome face, no matter what. I offered to cut my hair and have it made into a wig for him and he smiled a bit, but didn't really think he would look good as a strawberry blond, so I then offered Tim's hair because he has a lot of dark hair! (Sorry, Tim . . . thought you wouldn't mind!) Cryder gave him his nice knit UNC hat to wear, which he thinks he will just keep on his head from now on! We are off to UNC in a little while to watch them play Duke tonight. Always a big thrill for him to go back to college! Will write again soon. McNicey's off to put on her chauffeur hat!

    xoxoxox

Our days were scheduled around Lee's radiation treatments, but we also didn't want to miss Cryder's important games. The next one would be against Duke, UNC's nemesis. The radiologists were nice enough to change our appointments to first thing Wednesday morning and then late Thursday afternoon. That way we could leave right after radiation. I was crazed, trying to gather up all Lee's medications, food, and supplies for Cryder (bringing goodies to Cryder was a must!), and of course get my run in. If I was going to be stuck in the car for five hours, I had to get some exercise first or I'd be like a gerbil in a cage. This schedule meant getting up very early so I could fit everything in and still have time to send emails before I left.

Lee was particularly excited about this game. We had not beaten Duke in a while, and if there was one team Lee especially hated to lose to, it was Duke. The rivalry between the two teams was legendary. The really wonderful thing about this game, though, was that Cryder had been asked to be an honorary captain. Each week, the coach would choose a different team member to be the honorary captain, joining the two seasonal captains of the team. It was a huge honor, especially against Duke! It also meant Cryder had to make an inspirational speech to the team before the game, which is not an easy task for a somewhat quiet guy who shies away from the limelight.

We were driving to Chapel Hill again, which posed another challenge for us. The other thing torturing Lee was the massive size of the lump in his hamstring. It was painful all the time, and consequently it was almost impossible for him to find a comfortable way to sit. Car rides were the worst. There was no way for him to position himself so that he wasn't sitting on the lump.

Using one of the lessons I'd learned in my racing—coming up with solutions on the fly—I came up with the idea of making Lee a cushion. I bought a three-inch-thick square piece of foam rubber, held it up to the back of his leg and traced the area where the lump was protruding. I cut a hole out of the foam rubber to match the lump, and, presto, a perfect cushion for Lee. I suppose I could have covered it in fabric to make it look nicer, but it was simple and it worked!

The game started at 7 p.m., and it was a rainy, horrible night. I had come prepared for the weather, knowing how tough it would be for Lee to handle the rain and cold. So we were all bundled up and very excited to see Cryder walk out with the captains. I know Lee grew teary-eyed. I was all smiles, with my camera in hand. So proud of Cryder!

By half-time, Lee was shivering so much, though, that I was sure he wouldn't make it to the end of the game. Our friends were all passing blankets our way, but by the fourth quarter, the blankets were all wet and poor Lee was blue. I tried to convince him to go to the car and warm up—but no way was he leaving that game! I wrapped my arms around him and held him tight, trying to give him any warmth I had left, which wasn't much.

By the time the game ended, we didn't care if we were frozen or not. Carolina had beaten Duke for the first time in six years and eleven games and suddenly we were all charged up. Our boys were going wild. Jumping on each other and chanting—it was quite a sight. The boys played an amazing game. Despite the horrible, slanting rain, it was one of the best games I'd ever seen and one that we will never forget. When Cryder finally made his way over to the fence line, he was beaming. He was wet, dirty, and, unfortunately, wearing a mustache. All the guys had them . . . no shaving while they were on a winning streak. I later heard that Cryder's speech was incredible. Apparently, he spoke about his dad and the battle he was fighting. He wanted to win this for his dad. I heard the team was speechless after his talk. I would have been in tears.

The celebration after the game was going to be a good one. I was hoping Lee would be able to be a part of it. We had missed out on a lot of the celebrating so far, but maybe this night would be different. And celebrate we did. Lee even made it out to Top of the Hill for a nightcap (which, as his dutiful nurse, I drank for him).

But when morning came, Lee went from a high to a low. He'd gone to take a shower before we left, and I suddenly heard him gasp, and then say, "Oh my God."

"You all right?" I called in through the closed door.

He came out of the shower totally shaken up. His hair had fallen out in clumps and was all over the bathtub and all over the floor. I was devastated for him. "Here, come out," I said. "It's fine, you can't really tell, you still have a lot of hair. I'll clean it up."

The Carolina Inn was a beautiful historic hotel with wonderful cozy rooms. Our bathroom, though, was all tiled in white, so there was no hiding the black hair that lay everywhere. I quickly closed the door and got down on my hands and knees and gathered up the hair. I dumped it in the trash and hoped the cleaning ladies wouldn't be shocked.

On our car ride home, Lee was very quiet for a while. I let him be. He needed his space and this was one thing I couldn't fix anyway. After a while, he said he was going to call our friend "B" and ask him to drop off the buzz shears.

"Seriously?" I asked.

"Yes. That was the worst feeling this morning. Suddenly I was covered everywhere with my hair. It was going in my mouth and I couldn't breathe. It was awful. I can't do that again. I'm shaving my head."

I urged Lee to think about this again, as he still had a lot of hair and shaving his head would be an even more dramatic change.

"Why not just cut it really short, and that way you won't notice it as much when the hair falls out," I suggested. "It might be an easier transition. We can always shave it later. Baby steps!"

He agreed, and I know he felt better that once again he was controlling what he could. I sent out a quick email letting people know about Lee's hair so they wouldn't be shocked when they next saw him.

Of course Tim responded immediately, offering his hair in an amusing email that gave me a good laugh. I was cut short when a long-awaited email from Nurse Maureen popped up. My palms began sweating as I opened her email, but the news was a relief. The results from the blood tests came back NEGATIVE. Apparently, they'd concluded that Lee's red blood cells were so low from fighting the sarcoma, not from any other blood cancers. At least for now.

Friday afternoon, Lee had his last radiation treatment for that first round. It was a gorgeous day, so we decided to take a walk after his treatment. There was a beautiful park across from the doctor's office with a 7/8-mile asphalt path that surrounded the playing fields. We had fallen into a routine of walking in this park after Lee's radiation treatments. It was busy with children on bikes, walkers, runners, and kids playing lacrosse. There was always something to watch. It both entertained and distracted Lee, and more importantly, it allowed me to push him to walk a little further each time. By getting him to exert himself just a tad more every few days, he would keep his strength up, a technique that all my years of training and racing had taught me.

By the end of our walk we decided it was time to cut his hair, and I would be his hairdresser.

When we got home, I brought a stool from the kitchen outside and pulled out my haircutting scissors. I used to cut the boys' hair before they hit their teens and decided their parents didn't know how to do anything anymore. I still had the scissors in the kitchen drawer. Lee was waiting by the back door. "Don't worry, you are going to look so cute!" I assured him.

I cut it nice and short and swept the hair away as it fell so Lee wouldn't see it. I cut it down to about half an inch, and he looked very handsome—like a pilot, just like his father who used to fly for the air force. I sent him inside to look in the mirror to make sure it was as he wanted it. Not that I could glue it back on or anything. He was pleased, and I think very relieved that we didn't shave it. It was enough of a change.

We had a nice quiet weekend, readying ourselves for the second round of chemo. We were told that Hopkins would call on Sunday and confirm a bed for Monday morning. I guess they can never really rely on beds being available even though a date had been set. So by Sunday night, I began to worry and emailed our trusty Nurse Maureen, hoping she could work her magic. Unfortunately, we got word that they could not guarantee a bed and would call by noon on Monday to let us know if one was available. Ugh! Lee had been hoping to go down to Chapel Hill to watch Cryder's lacrosse game on Friday night. And I knew how important it was for him to look forward to something; to keep him motivated to stay strong enough to go. To make the game we'd have to leave Friday by noon, which meant he *had* to start chemo on Monday.

I wrote a quick note to Cryder:

Dad got bumped back a day on his room at Hopkins. He is very bummed. We sat around waiting for the call 'til 12:30 . . . no beds available, so we have to wait for tomorrow. Feel bad for Dad. He was anxious to get in and get started again. So we are home if you're looking for us. Xox

And Cryder wrote right back: "That's a total bummer. Tell him I'm sorry about that. I'll give you a call later on. Sitting in stupid class which I don't like but I just got one of my midterms back and got and 87 on it."

My response to Cryder and Tim: "He got a lollipop at radiation this morning for being a good boy!"

Tim's response: "Well, unless it was rum flavored, I think he is getting shafted!"

Thank goodness for my boys!

18

Staying Focused

The next couple of months contained more of the same. Two more rounds of chemo followed by radiation treatments. I was working hard doing what I could to keep up Lee's spirits, to be an advocate for him, to keep his routine as normal as possible. And in between treatments we attended Cryder's lacrosse games. Racing had given me both the confidence and discipline to demand what was fair when it came to making requests of the nurses and doctors, not to be overly self-centered, and to keep going in the face of all obstacles.

I was also trying very hard to keep Lee focused on the good things that were happening. It was essential for him to have a positive attitude; otherwise, he might be tempted to give up. I knew he was determined, but there were days when he struggled and it was hard to watch. By the end of March he'd lost a significant amount of weight too. Lee, a six-foot-one, well-proportioned man, had gone from 180 to 155, which made him look older and withered. Even scarier was the way Lee, who had always been so sharp and capable, just didn't have the energy to think or act for himself. I am quite sure he was unaware of how dependent he had become. I'm also sure that this was due in part to all the energy it took to fight the poison running through his body. I was, however, on top of the steps that had to be taken. My mind never seemed to shut down. When I hit the pillow at night, exhausted and so happy to be in my bed, my heavy eyelids would suddenly snap open, as I lay there wide-eyed, worrying about every second of what was to come.

After one trip to a lacrosse game without Lee, I arrived just in time for lunch and surprised him with a roast beef sandwich that I'd picked up at the deli en route. It was one of the few things he was able to eat that didn't taste awful. He wanted to hear every detail of Cryder's game; how the team had played, if I'd gotten a chance to needle his good friend about Princeton losing, and if Cryder was doing okay. I was happy to give him a very detailed report. I even returned with a little gift from Chapel Hill: a Tar Heel blue spiky wig to cover his balding head. He loved it and immediately put it on as we laughingly took pictures to send to friends.

I spent the rest of the day sitting with him as he drifted in and out. Clearly, the chemo was taking over again as his eyes appeared glassy and his lids grew heavy.

Before we knew it, though, we were back on the road to Chapel Hill. One of Lee's goals was to make it to Cryder's final home game on May 8, which was also senior day. Lee vowed he would attend that weekend event. I prayed that the surgery date would not conflict. I knew it would be close, but he just couldn't miss this.

Sent at the end of March:

Subject: Hospital escape!

Hi, Everyone. Sorry I haven't reported in a while. This is the first chance I've had to sit down and write since leaving Fri. morning for Chapel Hill. Here's why I had no time to write: I woke up at 5:20 a.m.; while drinking my LARGE mug of coffee, I packed up the brownies for the post game tailgate that I made at nine the night before, packed up McNicey's equipment (the IV flushes, alcohol wipes, shower patches, dressing changes, and the $3,000 (!) shot that had to be refrigerated and which I was to give him Sat. a.m.). I then raced to the pool and swam a mile and a half, raced home, folded laundry, ironed a few shirts, went for my 7-mile run, packed my and Lee's suitcases, showered and dried my hair, took out the garbage, packed up the car (including a pillow and blanket for my patient along with a bucket in case he got sick, and a "pee bottle" because he has to go to the bathroom every hour and we were NOT stopping every hour!!!!). I did all this by 9:30 a.m., with a stop at the bank, and was on my way to Hopkins to pick up Lee. I arrived to discover he'd had a terrible night, getting sick four times and no sleep. (Obviously the poor guy was not in great shape.) The nurse that was on duty, our favorite, was already getting the ball rolling to discharge him. Between the two of us, we had his stuff packed, got him showered, IVs removed and ready to go by the time the Dr's came in on rounds.

The only thing left was for Nurse Kavi to show me how to give Lee the shot on Sat. a.m. I was quite excited about a new procedure for McNicey. The nurse rolled up some gauze and wrapped it with tape . . . told me to hold the shot like a dart and punch it in at 90 degrees. My first time doing this . . . so a little nervous. I lined up the shot and jammed it into the gauze with Lee watching . . . He gave a little "ouch" when I stabbed too aggressively. Kavi winced a little and suggested a bit softer touch, and I gave it a few more practice tries and we were approved to leave.

In the elevator, it was just the two of us. I put his bag down and gave him a big hug and said, "Two down, one to go." The tears rolled down his cheeks and it reminded me of just how hard this was and how hard he was fighting. I got him settled into the back seat of the car for our five-hour drive. He slept most of the way (except through DC, where he said it was a little hard to sleep with my aggressive driving . . . a bit like a roller-coaster ride— imagine that??!!). I was on a mission to make it to Chapel Hill on time.

As we arrived in Chapel Hill, Lee started to stir in the back seat. He suddenly sat up in the back seat . . . eagerly looking out the window . . . beautiful spring day, flowers and trees blooming, and best of all for our patient . . . college students everywhere!! As we passed beautiful girls in sundresses and flip flops . . . my patient came to life! The game against Dartmouth was a perfect night, with the Heels winning once again. Next morning I gave Lee his shot. You will be very happy to hear that I performed my duty, as Lee said, "perfectly" and didn't hurt him at all. I do believe I have finally earned my nurse's hat!! Best to all of you and thanks for all your well wishes.

xox

A humorous response from Tim:

First point—Dad, I just wanted to say how amazing you are going through all this. We all knew you were a tough guy, but it really sounds like you are showing this treatment who's boss! Second point—Judging by the pace of this email and the description of Mom's daily life, I have concluded that she is clearly doing a lot of drugs, and I think as a family we all need to work to get her serious help!

Can't wait to see you guys this weekend!

Shortly after this, I wrote Dr. Frassica to find out when we needed to schedule surgery. I knew the timing meant it would be close to Cryder's final home game on May 8. The senior dinner following the game was traditionally when the dads would make their final speeches to their sons and Lee wanted to make his "father's speech" to his son in person. I also needed to know how many days he would be in the hospital post-surgery and whether he'd be on crutches or need a wheelchair. These were all things I was trying to prepare for. I also wanted to thank Dr. Frassica for the amazing team of doctors and nurses. We had not seen him since the day he told us about the sarcoma and I also wanted to let him know that Lee, despite the twenty-five pounds he'd lost, was handling the treatments pretty well.

Dr. Frassica responded immediately. We spent several days going back and forth with emails, trying to coordinate a day that all three doctors (Dr. Frassica, Dr. Attar, and the plastic surgeon) were available, plus Lee's skin still needed enough time to heal after the radiation. Radiated skin, if not given enough time, can lead to problems with infection and delayed healing after surgery. In the end, we set a date of May 10, which wasn't ideal for Lee because he wanted that lump out as quickly as possible, but he was willing to make the sacrifice so he could attend senior day. We had all learned to make sacrifices over the many years we'd been together.

I was also trying to stay on top of blood tests that were supposed to be scheduled, appointments with the chemo doctor, chest scans, and MRI's of his leg, all of which meant contacting Nurse Maureen. We had developed quite a friendship with all the nurses and doctors, and with each email they wanted updates on Lee—and the scores of the lacrosse games!

All my years of juggling training, racing, and mom duties had taught me to be extremely organized and prepare for what might be coming next. My skills were certainly coming in handy! I found that my days were zipping by, and I hardly had time to catch my breath. I was sleeping less and less but feeling optimistic overall.

Lee was amazing. He still insisted on going to work every morning during the weeks he had his radiation treatments. I would send him out the door with a bottle of Ensure in his pocket, just to make sure he was getting enough calories. He would come home around lunchtime, try to force down some food, and then take a nap before his afternoon radiation appointment. It was our new routine. After each session, we would drive across the street to the park and take our walk. Some days were harder than others, but he insisted. He wasn't going to give up. He was getting skinnier by the day, now folding his jeans over at the waist to keep them up. Everything was hanging off of him, and as much as I tried to entice him with his favorite foods, he wasn't interested.

We were seeing the light at the end of the tunnel. Only six radiation sessions left, then into Hopkins for his FINAL chemo treatment. Unfortunately, he had developed "thrush," a yeast infection on his tongue and throat, which is a common reaction to chemo. It caused a sour taste in his mouth though, and "nothing" tasted as it should, so the food that I put in front of him got pushed around his plate even more. I felt like I was back to the days of trying to make Tim eat his peas. Because Lee was still losing a lot of weight, I had to be a little tough on him. Ice cream, however, was now allowed any time of day! (By the end of his treatments in April, Lee weighed only 140 pounds!)

I had warned Tim and Gina that Lee had gotten very skinny and that almost all his hair was gone. Cryder had watched the changes weekly, but Tim and Gina hadn't seen him in more than a month. We had planned on meeting them for breakfast at the Carolina Inn, where we were all staying. We arrived first, and Lee went in to get a table. I waited for Tim and Gina by the hostess stand. Tim appeared around the corner, with a purposeful stride. I knew he was anxious to see his dad. He stopped to give me a hug, as did Gina. As we walked toward the table, Tim was looking around.

"Where is he?" he asked.

"Right there, right in front of you."

Lee had his back to us, and all Tim could see was a bald head on a very skinny body. Tim's shoulders dropped. But he quickly recovered and strode right over to give Lee a big hug. Though Tim didn't skip a beat, I knew he did not expect to find his father looking like that. In Tim's typical fashion, he made light of the situation and Lee was all smiles, as was I.

Cryder snuck in for a few minutes before his big game against the University of Maryland to be with us. You can imagine how happy Lee was to have both his boys and Gina surrounding him.

I know it's been a week since I wrote. I don't know where the time goes, but it seems to fly by. We had a great time in Chapel Hill last weekend. Game day was the most beautiful Carolina day with blue skies and temps in the seventies. The stands were packed and the game was a battle between UNC and MD, both undefeated teams in the top five. Luckily for everyone's weekend . . . UNC won and life was good in Chapel Hill! Tim and Gina joined us at half time . . . somehow Tim had a hard time navigating his way along Franklin Street. He claimed he was ambushed by the alums who were down for the weekend and forced into the bars. As much as Gina tried . . . he kept escaping! However, he was a VERY enthusiastic fan to make up for missing the first half!

It was a long day for Lee, with the game starting at two. Of course, we had to go to our usual watering/celebrating spot after the game and sit on the porch at P-Bobs. By the time we got to dinner, Lee was really wiped out and after dinner we went back to our room while the rest of the gang went out to celebrate a big win. It was killing him not to go and I could see the sadness in his eyes. But it was a good day nonetheless.

Today UNC is arriving in Baltimore to play Hopkins. We are hosting the team for dinner and it is supposed to be eighty and sunny for the whole weekend! Cryder is allowed to stay after the game and we are so excited to have him home. Hope you all have a wonderful Easter. We are on the downside of the roller-coaster hill!! Best to all of you and please keep the positive thoughts going.

xoxox

The end was getting closer!

The team dinner I'd been planning and was responsible for turned out to be a big success and we loved having the boys—they were always so gracious! Lee was all smiles as each player made a point of shaking his hand and thanking us for such a nice dinner. The game was even better with UNC remaining undefeated by beating Hopkins!

19

The End . . . of a Sort

There is the saying, "All good things must come to an end," but bad things end, too, and Lee was about to endure the last of his treatments. We were both feeling a little more optimistic. Lee had made it through some tough days and nights with the end now in sight. We would celebrate that and look forward to our plans for the next month before surgery.

The heart of Cryder's lacrosse season was coming up with the highly anticipated UNC vs. UVA game at the Meadowlands in New Jersey. We had a big group of friends and family meeting at the Meadowlands, many of whom were coming not only to watch Cryder play in such an exciting venue but to see Lee and celebrate his completion of treatment. But there were still hurdles to jump, and I couldn't let down my guard yet.

I went with Lee, as I always did, to his radiation treatment. Because it was his last treatment, his doctor wanted to check the lump, and when she had Lee turn his back and pull down his pants, I was shocked at the mass that had seemingly expanded in the last week. I'm sure my eyes widened with fear and I caught my breath, but didn't want to scare Lee, so I kept silent.

With his treatments finished, we hugged and thanked all the nurses and Dr. Frassica, saying goodbye and hoping to never return. They loved Lee and wished him well, his charm always winning people over. Then we sped off to Hopkins to finish the last chemo. Despite my fear of this lump, I couldn't help but be somewhat excited that we were approaching the end.

However, my fears came back to haunt me when I lay in bed that night, with images of this horrible tumor growing out of Lee's leg. I tossed and turned and finally got out of bed at 5 a.m. and sent an email to Dr. Frassica, sharing my fears at the size of Lee's seemingly growing lump. I instantly felt a weight had been lifted, knowing I was at least alerting his doctors of my concerns.

I had to rid myself of the nervous energy pent up with a quick run, which always seemed to remind me of the power and strength I had within. When I returned feeling cleansed and ready to face the day, I sat at my usual spot by the computer writing and checking emails. I was calmed to read a reply from Dr. Frassica saying that he would check on Lee first thing this morning. I could breathe freely now.

I had to leave Lee for twenty-four hours and fly to Florida to close our apartment after the renters left. I hated to leave him but the only time I could go was when he was in the hospital with others to care for him. When I arrived in Florida I got a call from Lee, who excitedly told me about a visit from Dr. Frassica. I hadn't told Lee about my email to Dr. Frassica, and my fears about his lump, so I played along acting surprised to hear about the visit. He said the doctors were very positive and went over what the procedure would be and what he should expect. When I returned on Wednesday morning, Lee still seemed to be on a high and it warmed my heart to see the big smile on his face when I entered his room. Of course, you couldn't see my smile through the surgeon's mask I had to wear, which I quickly pulled away to sneak in a kiss!

I settled into my chair next to Lee's bed for the rest of the day. It was 7:30 p.m. when the last bag of chemo was almost empty. I was fixated on Lee's chemo drip for the last hour. As it counted down and clicked away with each drip, I was watching. I wanted to witness that last drip and say, "There, you didn't beat us! We are strong and fighting!" I say "we" with a little hesitance because it had been Lee doing most of the fighting. But we had been a team, and I had given him everything I had within me to help him battle. I only wish I could do more to take his pain away.

We had been told that the chemo tends to make you more emotional. Lee has always been one who isn't afraid to show his tears. Not that he is wimpy, but there have been things that set him off. Just mention the movie *Brian's Song*, for instance, and his eyes well up! I love that about him. When the chemo was finishing the last drips, Lee was watching too. It was a moment that is ingrained in my mind. I don't think he expected such a wave of emotion to hit him, but it did. And only he knows how tough the last few months really were. I just wanted to hug him forever!

I had so many responses to Lee's final chemo report; some emotional ones from my sisters and brother, telling me how much they admired both of us for our strength, our fighting spirit, and what an inspiration Lee is. There was one email from my aunt who apologized for being remiss and not writing before, but I assured her there were no hurt feelings. I found it interesting, throughout this illness, that cancer is a scary thing and everyone handles it differently. Some shy away, not sure how to speak of cancer, and some people you hardly know are on your doorstep offering help in any way. We were lucky to have so many that cared and a family that never ceased to amaze me. And we were looking forward to seeing a huge group of friends and family all uniting in Meadowlands the day after Lee would be released from Hopkins after his final chemo. We just had to get there!

And get there we did, despite a terrible morning of Lee being nauseous, we drove into the meadowlands parking lot to find our UNC family with a great big UNC Lacrosse banner flying high. There were big smiles and welcoming cheers as Lee climbed out of the car. The game was thrilling, despite the loss to UVA, and Cryder beamed when he saw his father wave from the stands.

Just when I thought we had everything planned perfectly, we were thrown another curveball. They had to move the surgery up a week to May 3, which meant Lee would only have five days to recover to make it to Cryder's final home lacrosse game and the senior dinner. That only worried me a little because in the two weeks after Lee had finished his last radiation and chemo treatments he'd begun showing signs of his old self. As his "coach," I told him that he really needed to focus on gaining back some strength and muscle before going into surgery. I compared it to training for an Ironman: when you enter the final period, it's time to rebuild and get stronger by race day. Each day he walked, with me marching at his side, urging him on, following our old route along a stream at the edge of the woods.

A few more lacrosse games, some wins, and a couple of disappointments, and we arrived to the week before Lee's surgery. Everything seemed to be going very well. In the meeting with Dr. Attar, he showed us a scan of Lee's tumor, which was far larger than what we'd imagined. Previously we'd only known its dimensions. Seeing it was a bit of a shock. But Dr. Attar was concerned by how close to the sciatic nerve it was.

One slight mistake and Lee might lose sensation in parts of his leg and foot, and even worse, he might have to wear a brace for the rest of his life. I briefly tried to imagine my active husband dealing with that. But Dr. Attar expressed confidence that it wouldn't be affected, which we very much hoped, but then, as always, things were put into perspective for us when he let us know that his number one priority was to save Lee's life.

He described the incision. It would be long, running from the middle of Lee's butt to below the middle of his thigh. As we left the appointment, Lee turned to Dr. Attar, who is young and very professional, and said, "See you bright and early (5:30 a.m.) on Monday . . . I'm counting on you; no partying for you this weekend!"

Dr. Attar looked at him quite seriously and said, "I'm counting on me too!"

The weekend before the surgery was supposed to be beautiful, and Lee hoped to get in a little golf. Both boys had said they would come to Hopkins on Monday, but I told them to stay put and promised to keep them updated hourly. But Tim insisted on coming anyway. He didn't want me sitting in the hospital, waiting alone, and he wanted to be there for his dad, too. Tim has a very big heart! He bought himself a train ticket that would have him arriving in Baltimore by six o'clock. Lee was going to be so surprised, I thought; it would mean the world to him that Tim was there, and me too!

By Friday, I felt that everything was in place. I had checked and double-checked the details of the surgery, and it was all set. As far as Lee was concerned, there was only one more thing left to do. He had made an appointment with our lawyer to go over our wills. It made me think of the first time we left Tim when he was a baby, flying south for a long weekend. Three nights before we left, I woke up in a panic in the middle of the night, shook Lee awake, and told him we had to make a will before we left. I am sure he thought I was overreacting, but he appeased me anyway. Now, I did the same for him. He needed the peace of mind that everything was taken care of.

It turned out to be a gorgeous weekend. Our usual routine was to get our exercising and yard work or errands done during the morning and, after lunch, go walk nine holes on the golf course. Yes, he was walking nine holes and proud of it! The Kentucky Derby was on Saturday and I wanted to be back in time to watch. In my next life, I would love to come back as a racehorse. I had given Tim a call before leaving for golf to check in. I knew Gina was in DC for the weekend on business, and Tim was out on Long Island with the boys.

I hated when he was with the boys and without Gina. Lee gave me a hard time for worrying about him, reminding me that Tim was twenty-six years old and a grown man now. He was right, but I knew Tim! When I called that Saturday afternoon, Tim answered his phone quickly because he was headed out to play golf, too, and couldn't be on his cellphone. He promised to call back later.

We had a great time playing golf and then raced home to watch the Derby. Life was good. Tim, of course, forgot to call back, but my mother happened to go to the club for dinner and ran into Tim and his friends watching the Derby in the men's bar. Figures! She loved it when she ran into Tim, and relished even more being able to call to tell me she'd seen him, making me jealous! He was having fun, as he always did.

Early morning on Sunday I went for a good long hour-and-a-half run, knowing I would be sitting in the hospital for most of Monday. We decided to get golf in before lunch so that Lee could have the afternoon to rest and get things ready to go to the hospital. We were home by twelve thirty. Again, it was a gorgeous day and a perfect day for lunch outside.

I checked voicemails hoping to hear from Tim, but his phone went straight to voicemail, so either he had turned it off or it had lost its charge. I was starting to get that "worried mom" thing when Lee came into the kitchen and told me to stop it.

"He is fine. Why are you pestering him?"

What Lee didn't understand was that I had a nagging feeling that something was about to go wrong with Tim, or already had. Finally, at one o'clock, the phone rang. It was Tim.

"Where the heck have you been? I've been trying to reach you since yesterday. You know how worried I get when Gina's not around to keep an eye on you!"

"Oh, stop your worrying! I am fine, Mother," he said lightheartedly.

Someday, when they have their own children, my boys will understand what it's like to worry—although I don't think men worry nearly as much as women, because they let us do most of the worrying for them! So Tim was fine, and Cryder was studying for exams, and it was a lovely Sunday. We were all fine, and soon Lee would be free of this lump.

We lounged out by the pool for a while and puttered around. I did some yard work, while Lee started to pack his things. It was three thirty when the phone rang again. It was Tim's cell phone, only this time it wasn't Tim.

"Mrs. D, it's Max."

With his next words, my whole world fell apart.

20

The Crash

Tim had been staying at Max's house near Glen Cove on the North Shore of Long Island for the weekend. Without Gina there to rein Tim in, there were bound to be boys doing the stupid things boys do. Call it mother's intuition, but I'd sensed trouble. When I answered the phone the second time that Sunday afternoon and saw Tim's caller ID, I was laughing to myself, thinking I'd really made him feel guilty for not calling and now he was making up for it. Tim is a very in-touch kind of guy. It's not at all unusual for him to call several times a day when something pops into his head that he wants to share with me. The age of cell phones!

When it was Max's voice on Tim's phone, my heart sank. I knew something was wrong. I heard Max's words—"there's been an accident"—but processed them in slow motion. I had been on a high, with Lee's surgery finally less than twenty-four hours away. Then suddenly this call. I felt as though someone had kicked my legs out from under me and was sitting on my chest. I couldn't breathe. Fear pumped through me with each beat of my heart. *Oh, Tim, what have you done?*

Since he was a little boy, I was constantly saying, "Tim, don't do that." Most of the time he would do it anyway, and something would happen. He would come to me with an incredibly sad face, alligator tears brimming in his eyes, and say, "Sorry, Mom. I messed up." He pulled at my heartstrings. And he always seemed. very upset with himself for disappointing us.

Tim had been diagnosed with ADD when he was a child, and I partly blamed his impulsiveness on that, but it was also just Tim. He was a constant worry. But it was in high school that he really scared me, and his father, too. He had two terrible car accidents, one when he was the passenger and the other as the driver. Both times I had warned him: Do not do anything stupid tonight. Please be careful and make good decisions. "Okay, okay, Mom. Don't you know I'm invincible?" Mostly, that's the way our conversations went. Don't most high school boys think like that?

In the first accident, I don't know how either boy walked away unhurt after the car flipped over the barrier on the highway, landing sideways against oncoming traffic. The second accident was in the spring of his senior year. Tim was driving, and thank God he was alone when his car hit a telephone pole because the impact destroyed the passenger side of his car. Again, he was spared. I warned him that he was running out of luck.

As a junior in college, Tim went to London for a summer internship. It was July, and the rest of our family was in Delray. Early one morning Cryder was still sleeping and I was enjoying my coffee. I turned on the TV to catch up on the news. The coverage from London was saying that the subways (the famous Tube) had been bombed. As I watched in horror, Lee came in for his coffee and saw the TV, too.

"Please tell me that's not on Tim's subway line," I pleaded.

Lee's eyes opened wide. "Yes, it is. He goes through King's Cross Station right about this time."

For hours we couldn't reach Tim. We were terrified. To make matter worse, the cell phone systems were shut down out of fear that it was how the terrorists detonated the bombs.

We finally reached Tim and found out he had been one stop from King's Cross when the bomb exploded, a matter of minutes away. He was fine, but obviously quite shaken. I wanted him to come home. But not Tim. The approaching weekend was the highlight of his summer. He had plans to go skydiving in Sweden!

I pleaded with him to reconsider his plans, after all, he had just barely missed being bombed in the London underground—did he really need to go throw himself out of a perfectly good airplane? In Tim's usual manner—because he always seems to have an answer for everything—he said, "Mom, you can't let things like that run your life. You never know when you won't be here anymore. You have to live your life and follow your dreams."

Well, true, but I was a little skeptical about the necessity of launching oneself out of a plane!

I tried to make sense of what Max was saying. Tim had broken both his legs and lost a lot of blood, he explained, but he was conscious and "okay." His brief description raised countless other questions: How much blood? How had he broken both legs? If he was okay then why couldn't we speak to him, and so on.

He ended by saying that the paramedics were loading Tim into a helicopter—*a helicopter!?*—and that Sara, Max's girlfriend, had called Gina, but she was still on the train approaching New York.

"They're airlifting Tim to the Nassau University Medical Center," he said, which I knew was a facility in the middle of Long Island. "I'm on my way there," he added. He'd call again once he arrived.

Lee was in the kitchen, listening in on the conversation. We were both in shock. I started to cry, and he came to my side and held me. While we were desperate to know more, maybe it was best that for the moment our information remained sketchy. Had we known the full extent of Tim's injuries we would have been even more devastated and worried.

For several minutes after Max's call neither Lee nor I knew what to do. Then we sprang into action, making calls. I phoned Jack, my stepfather, who dropped everything and raced to the hospital, calling from his car phone to get directions as he drove. Fortunately, the facility was the local shock trauma hospital; in other words, the best place for someone who'd been in a bad accident to be taken to. At the same time, I phoned Gina on the train, but she was trapped there until the station. She was frantic.

I called Mom, too, who drove like a madwoman from Connecticut to get to Tim. But then her car started smoking and she got stuck on the Throgs Neck Bridge in bumper-to-bumper traffic. She called us in a panic, and Lee told her to get out of the car. She called back a few minutes later and told us it was fine now, that traffic was moving and she was going straight to the hospital.

"Are you sure it's fine?" I asked. "You probably can't see the smoke because you're moving!" But in typical fashion, nothing would stop her; she was going to get to that hospital.

A while later, we got the initial medical report from Max. He said that Tim had broken both legs very badly, but he knew little else. We still weren't sure how much he was telling us but understood that the accident was very serious. Chaotic thoughts ran through our minds. All we wanted was for our son to survive and to figure out the very best treatment options for him. With relatively little information to work on, we decided Tim should be transported to the Hospital for Special Surgery in New York City, where we knew one of the doctors. Just as we were about to embark on a series of calls to make that happen, we received a call from one of Tim's doctors—a trauma surgeon in the ER—to whom we mentioned that we thought Tim should be moved.

Without any emotion at all, he told us that Tim was in very bad shape, that under no circumstances could he be moved, and that they were working to save his leg, which had been very badly damaged. Though the doctor didn't say it directly, he implied that Tim had been so severely injured that his life was actually at stake.

When I heard this my own legs went weak and I left the room. I couldn't believe this was happening and couldn't hold back my fears *or* my tears. In the kitchen, Lee was still speaking to the doctor, somehow managing to keep his tone calm.

"Thank you," he said. "I am so sorry. Please go and do whatever you can to save his leg and his life."

His life? I thought. *Oh, my God!* Then Lee hung up and came around the corner to soothe me. In that moment I felt as if we were reversing roles. Now he was taking care of me after I'd been taking care of him for several months, trying to be his rock in every way, but with this added on top of everything else, I simply broke down.

"Oh, God, I knew it, I just knew it. What do we do?" I said, my mind reeling with worst-case scenarios. "Should we drive up there?"

At this point I was crying uncontrollably. Lee reminded me that Jack and Mom were there and that they would do what was needed. But I wanted to go too, and had trouble thinking clearly. *This was my child; my boy. How could we go up there when Lee's long-awaited surgery was taking place in less than thirteen hours? Could I go up there alone and leave Lee? No, no, no, I couldn't.*

While I went on in this manner, Lee was able to tap into his own reservoir of strength. I can only imagine that the danger Tim was in made Lee forget his own imminent surgery and focus completely on his son. In any case, he now had the strength to hold me until I calmed down.

It was going to be a long night. My poor Tim—he was fighting for his life. I walked around the house in a daze, watching the phone, willing it to ring. I kept praying over and over: *Please, God, oh, please let him keep his leg. Please save him.*

What we later found out was that Tim had been the passenger in an off-road vehicle called a Gator, a type of four-wheel all-terrain utility vehicle. He and a friend, David, had been racing along paths through a wooded area surrounding Max's house, travelling at speeds of up to 35 mph. At once, the ATV flew over a bump. David lost control and suddenly they were headed into a tree with the passenger side of the vehicle about to take the brunt of the crash. Tim tried to exit, but his legs got caught in the cab of the Gator, which sheared the skin, as well as significant amounts of tissue and muscle, off of the lower part of his left leg, leaving the tibia completely exposed. When he landed, both legs faced the wrong direction and blood was everywhere. Dirt filled the wounds with debris, which was very serious because of the high probability of infection.

Despite all this, Tim remained conscious. On seeing his destroyed left leg, he somehow had the presence of mind to use his belt as a tourniquet to stanch the flow of blood, and he managed to hand his cell phone to David, who was physically okay but acting hysterical. Tim calmly told him to call 911. Max had gone to the train station a few miles away when the accident happened and arrived back at his house just as the paramedics arrived.

Hours passed as Lee and I waited to hear more from the doctors. It wasn't until seven o'clock that I suddenly realized we hadn't called Cryder. He was horrified at the news and said he was coming right home. The last thing I wanted to worry about was Cryder driving for five hours from Chapel Hill late at night. "Stay put," I told him. "We'll call the minute we hear anything. There's nothing you can do and you have exams tomorrow and playoffs."

The doctors didn't call until ten forty-fve that night. They were out of surgery. They'd saved Tim's leg, but he was very clear that Tim was not out of the woods yet. He had broken his left leg in three places, two compound fractures on the tibia and one on the femur that was not as bad. He'd also broken the right tibia. The reason for all the blood loss, he explained, was because of the major artery that had been severed in his left leg.

Undoubtedly there were other surgeries ahead, and infection was a huge concern. There was also a likelihood of nerve damage that they wouldn't know about until the swelling went down and he could test whether he still had feeling in his foot. Walking could be an issue and he might have to have a brace. More importantly Tim was still at risk of losing his left leg.

Though my mother didn't say this to us, she was terrified when she first saw Tim. His skin tone was yellowish gray and he looked as though death were fast approaching. And the fact was, death was still stalking him.

Lee and I finally dragged ourselves to bed around twelve thirty in the morning, knowing we had to get some sleep before leaving for

Hopkins at 5 a.m. Lee especially needed his strength for the operation. As soon as my head hit the pillow, however, the demons started racing through my mind. My eyes snapped open and I stared at the ceiling. The thoughts about Tim and Lee were terrifying. By the time I'd dozed off, the calls began coming.

Phone calls in the middle of the night are always startling, but on this night to receive one at 2 a.m. shot me out of bed. The voice at the other end was Cryder's. He didn't want to frighten us by barging in and was letting us know he was about to arrive. He said he could not have sat still in Chapel Hill waiting for a call to hear about his brother and about his father's surgery. He had to be with us. He said he was here to take care of his father and I should go to Tim. I was so incredibly grateful he didn't listen when I told him to stay in Chapel Hill.

A couple of hours later, when Lee and I got in the car to drive to Hopkins, we discussed what to do about Tim. Now that Cryder was here and would be at his side, Lee urged me to go to Long Island after he was out of surgery. To myself I thought, *If everything goes well, I'll drive straight to the hospital in Long Island.* So strange the way both of our fears had shifted away from Lee's surgery and now were focused on Tim. It all seemed like a terribly bad dream, and I wondered how we would fight our way out of it.

21

Two Patients—One Stable, One Critical

It wasn't long before they took Lee to prep him for surgery. I was in the waiting room, again, watching the clock. It was still too early to make calls to my family to see if they had any news on Tim. I figured no news was good news, and though my body sat there, my mind was elsewhere.

Around 7:30 a.m., I received a call from a friend to check on me, and when I glanced up in mid sentence, there was my mother standing in front of me.

"Oh my God! Mom! What are you doing here?" I burst into tears, and threw myself into her arms.

"Did you really think I was going to let you sit here alone? I couldn't let you do that, not with what you're going through," she said, tears brimming in her eyes.

"How did you get here?" I asked. She'd booked herself on the first flight out of Long Island and somehow found me at Hopkins, a feat in itself! She planned to bring me back home with her to be with Tim. She had tickets on a flight around three o'clock. I was so grateful to her. For a few minutes, my body relaxed and I felt safe.

I think she tried to minimize how badly Tim looked, and instead reminded me that he was a young, strong guy. "He's going to fight through this," she said. Then, as we waited to hear how Lee's surgery was going, my friend Ruth Anne unexpectedly arrived. She hadn't heard about Tim and when she did, she was devastated. She knew Tim almost as well as her own children.

She then told me some more bad news. Her son Austin and Cryder were the best of friends growing up, and even now they had a big group of high school pals who'd all remained very close. One of the girls who was about to graduate from the University of Virginia, had suffered a tragic death in the early hours of May 3, apparently killed by her ex-boyfriend. The story was unbelievable and incredibly sad. I wondered, briefly, why so many bad things seemed to be happening at once.

Cryder arrived at the hospital around noon and looked exhausted, too. When I asked him if he knew what had happened at UVA, his shoulders drooped and his eyes were cast down.

"Yes," he said. "I got the call in the car driving up here, but I didn't want to tell you and upset you even more." Poor guy. He was hurting too, and yet there was nothing I could do to fix things for him.

Finally, Dr. Frassica appeared in the waiting room. With a big smile on his face, he said that everything had gone well. The tumor, though, was much bigger than we'd expected. Dr. Attar held up his hands to show me its size, which shocked me. He said he had to remove a lot of muscle and tissue surrounding the tumor, which meant that Lee had a huge incision, but that he'd be able to walk fine and gain his strength back with therapy. We were so grateful and relieved.

I told Dr. Frassica about Tim and that I intended to leave right after I saw Lee in recovery. He asked for the name of the hospital and the doctor, pulled out his cell phone and called. He spoke with Tim's doctor and asked all sorts of questions. When he hung up, he said that he felt Tim was in good care, but that he had suffered quite an injury. Somehow his words were reassuring at just the right moment.

Shortly thereafter, I went to see Lee, who was still clearly under the clouds of anesthesia, but he could see and hear me. I leaned over and kissed him.

"You did great," I told him. "They got the tumor, it's all gone. And the sciatic nerve wasn't touched. You're going to be fine."

Now it was his turn to shed some tears. I kept wiping them away while he kept groggily asking, "So the tumor is all gone?"

"Yes," I said. Then I told him Mom had flown down and had a ticket for me to go see Tim.

"Yes," he said. "Go take care of Tim. Tell him I love him."

Mom and I drove from the airport and stopped at a CVS pharmacy about fifteen minutes from the hospital where Jack was meeting us to take Mom home, leaving me with her car. I ran into CVS to grab a toothbrush and when I came out Jack was there getting out of the car to give me a hug. He had spent much of the day at the hospital watching over Tim.

"Listen, kiddo," he said very seriously, "you need to be prepared. Tim has had a rough time. He looks pretty bad."

I took a deep breath, understanding he was willing me to be strong. Looking deep into his blue eyes that held my gaze I accepted his transfer of strength. "Okay," I said, "Okay."

I couldn't drive fast enough to the hospital. It was supposedly the top emergency hospital in the area and handled most of the horrific accidents on the highways of Long Island. I later found out that it was also attached to a prison, which explained the very bare, dreary lobby and the armed guard at the front desk.

I found my way to the ICU. The doors opened, and I steadied myself as I rounded the corner. I was walking toward the curtained beds and thought I saw someone who vaguely resembled Tim with a few people standing by his bed, their backs to me. But that patient was so bloated and swollen that I couldn't imagine it was him.

I asked a nearby nurse where I might find Tim DiPietro. She looked up and pointed at the patient I'd been looking at. It *was* him. As I drew nearer to his bed, I could see his mouth taped closed with a tube down his throat (he was on a respirator), and then suddenly Gina turned and saw me. The woman next to her was her mom, and her dad was there, too.

"Tim, Tim," Gina was saying. "Look! Your Mom's here!"

My throat tightened and tears welled up in my eyes. Tim couldn't talk because of the respirator, but his eyes said everything. He also had a pad and pen and wrote in big looping letters, *sorry mom*. He was blaming himself for the accident and for putting us through even more heartache.. Then tears began running down both our cheeks.

"It's okay, Tim. I love you." I hugged him as best I could, trying to avoid disturbing all the tubes and IV lines attached to him. We were all crying now and holding on to each other around Tim's curtained bed.

As soon as I could compose myself, I told Tim how much Cryder and Dad loved him. Tim kept writing: *I love you, I'm sorry*. Then he added: *Dad?? I'm so happy you're here*.

"I know you are. It's Okay. I love you too," and as I leaned in close and stroked his arm, I continuedto tell him his father was going to be just fine and had sent all his love.

I called Lee and Cryder at the Hopkins Medical Center, who both got on the phone. When Tim heard his Dad's voice, tears started streaming again. I could hear Lee saying, "I love you, Tim. Be strong." Tim was nodding yes, while I was wiping away his tears, and mine.

Tim was in very rough shape, though initially I saw little except the sheets that covered him up to his chest. Underneath I saw that his legs were heavily bandaged, and a pump extended from one of them. It was filling a large plastic container at the end of his bed with a bloody fluid, presumably something draining from his wound. He was surrounded by monitors, numerous IVs, and bags of fluid hanging from metal poles like Lee's IV pole, Stanley. With all the equipment there was just enough room for a couple of people to stand at either side of his bed, and one or two at the end.

On a lighter note, at one point the doctor came around and Tim wrote: *Mobility? Damage? How long? When can I ski?* Thank God for his spirit! The doctor explained he'd be going in for another surgery the next day to try to clean the wound some more. They also planned to "rod" his leg, but not until the infection was under control.

Around eight o'clock, the doctors suggested that we let Tim rest. Seeing how torn Gina and I were, they assured us that he would be closely watched (his bed was right across from the nurses' station) and that they would call us if anything became worrisome. I kissed Tim and told him to get some sleep, that we had to go but would be back first thing in the morning. He nodded that he understood. His big blue eyes looked deep into mine. Poor Gina could hardly tear herself away.

Despite my exhaustion I had trouble sleeping. I felt like I was floating through a movie, watching someone else's life. It seemed like days had passed since Max's phone call. Finally, I got out of bed, went down on my knees and, with my hands clasped together, I leaned against the bed and prayed to God, again. *Please, oh please, don't take Tim, don't take his leg. Please, God, let Tim and Lee be okay.* I said it over and over until I think I finally fell asleep that way. It was another terrible night, with very little sleep. I kept expecting my phone to ring at any moment. Thank goodness, it remained silent.

At a time like this, I'm not sure there are any racing lessons you can rely on to get you through. What helped, though, and what we were incredibly grateful for, were all the people who provided their support to Lee and me, in one form or another, in the weeks leading up to Tim's horrific accident, and then even more so in the aftermath. We'd been close to feeling some relief that we'd conquered Lee's tumor, that his cancer was gone. To have a son then hovering on the brink of death was, plain and simple, every parent's nightmare. And I wondered if I truly had the reserves necessary to pull us through this next race.

22

Tim—After the Crash

My plan, if you could call it that, was to go back to the hospital Tuesday morning, and, if Tim was doing better, I would race back to Baltimore later in the day to be with Lee.

When Gina, Mom, and I got to the hospital Tuesday morning, however, things were not looking good at all. We were hoping to find Tim more alert. That was not the case. He seemed disoriented and distant, almost as if he were slipping away.

I noticed the pad of paper on Tim's table where he'd been writing messages and questions the day before. It was open to a page that was scribbled with large writing. *Is my mom or girlfriend still here?* Next page: *I can't breathe. Normal?* Next page: *Scared.*

Tears filled my eyes, and Gina's too. Why hadn't I insisted on staying in the hospital for the night? How could I have left him? I know Gina was feeling the same.

As Tim's friends started to filter in, their faces said it all. His best childhood friend, Coly was first to arrive. He was clearly shocked, and I could see him struggling, trying to think of something to say. As he spoke, Tim was trying hard to find the face that matched the voice, but his eyes seemed to be focusing on something far beyond where we stood. I spoke softly, telling Tim that Coly was here to visit, hoping he could identify him, but at the same time I was terrified, not sure how to make sense of his behavior.

A nurse informed us that Tim was scheduled for another surgery around three o'clock to clean out the wound and remove dead tissue. But was he strong enough to withstand anesthesia and another surgery? I would discuss it with one of the doctors; I had already decided there was no way I could leave Tim's side. Though I also wanted to be with Lee, he would have to rely on our friends in Baltimore. They had rallied around him and were taking turns visiting him at the hospital. I was reluctant to break the news to him, not just that I wasn't coming home, but also that Tim seemed in bad shape. And I would have to tell him soon.

A number of Tim and Gina's friends came by and offered us food, drinks, and a chance to take a break. They were truly wonderful, this group of friends from Tim's childhood, who he'd reconnected with when he'd moved up to Manhattan. But neither Gina nor I wanted to leave his bedside. So we didn't; instead, we, along with his friends, rotated in and out of the small room, each of us lending support to the other.

Cell phone service was terrible in the ICU. But cell service from one hospital to the next was even worse, making it almost impossible to talk with Lee and Cryder. I was relieved to hear how well Lee sounded. They were going to get him up to walk later that day. I was happy for him and put on my strongest, most determined voice and told them that Tim would pull through. I was trying hard to sound positive, and certainly wanted to believe that would be the case.

When my phone rang again, it was my father. When I heard "Tigs, it's Dad," I began to sob and couldn't stop. My relationship with my father was complicated—a novel in itself—but just hearing him call me Tigs, the nickname he'd given me as a child because I never stopped bouncing around like Tigger in *Winnie-the-Pooh*, meant so much. He wanted to know where we were and what was going on. I struggled to regain my composure, but all I could say was: "Oh, Dad, I don't know, I don't know . . . he's in bad shape. I'm so scared."

After my father married his third wife and established another life, we saw less and less of each other—not for lack of trying on my part. Despite his lack of communication and the hurt feelings I had over the years from his neglect, in my eyes he still could do no wrong. Whenever he called, I came running. Hearing his voice in the ICU that day broke down one of the walls I'd so carefully constructed. Add to that the lack of sleep, and I'm not sure what I was crying about. Everything, I suppose: my relationship with my father, my inability to be in two places at once, and most of all my worry about Tim. I didn't know how many more tears I had, but here they were again. And the worst of the afternoon was yet to come.

As the day wore on, Tim was growing less and less responsive. I noticed, though, that he always seemed more alert when Dr. Noel came by to check on him. She'd been the one who'd talked to us the previous night when Tim was writing questions about skiing. She had told him about her husband, a soccer player who had injured his legs in a terrible accident. The outlook had not been good, but he'd fought through it and was back on his feet doing well. Her story gave Tim hope.

In a weak moment, I went to find her, too. I was in tears and apologized. I explained about Lee and said I hoped she understood why I was such a mess. I just needed to know, was Tim going to make it, was he going to live? She nodded yes, and put her arms around me and told me not to apologize. "Tim will be OK," she said. I trusted her and somehow felt some comfort.

There was a patient next to Tim, separated by a white curtain, whose name was Mr. Lee. He was in really bad shape, too. As much as you tried to ignore it, you could hear everything going on. He seemed to be in and out of consciousness. The nurses were constantly coming to his bedside, and in raised voices, they called his name, "Mr. Lee, Mr. Lee." Every time Tim heard that, he would open his eyes and look around. He still wasn't seeing clearly, but I think he was looking for Lee. In his cloudy world, he probably thought his dad was there and someone was calling his name.

It's funny how you can stand by a hospital bed for hours and hours (there were no chairs) and not feel your legs getting tired. They just go numb, like the rest of you. Time goes by, but because there are no windows in the ICU you have no idea what time of day it is or what's going on in the outside world. It doesn't matter. There is continual activity around you, with buzzers and bells going off constantly. There are patients who are quiet and ones in obvious agony. Family members and friends shuffle through, trying to respect your privacy and not invade your space.

At one point, there was an awful wail four beds down. It startled me, and I looked up to see a woman collapsing to her knees. I knew what had happened; so heart-wrenching. All I could think was, *Please, oh, please don't let that happen to us.*

I hadn't met Tim's lead doctor yet, so when Dr. Routolo came by to see us at two o'clock, I was anxious to talk to him. He was very businesslike and got right to the point. That was good. I wanted him to be direct and honest. He explained Tim's situation and the surgery that afternoon. The wound was very dirty and needed to be cleaned. Tim had also lost a great deal of blood, and a lot of dead tissue had to be removed.

After he left, I tried to tell Tim that he was going in for another surgery and that we would all be nearby in the waiting room, but I wasn't sure he heard me. At two fifteen they wheeled him away as we all stood and watched, each of us silently praying, I'm sure.

We waited for a report in that small waiting room, just big enough for the seven of us. Max went to get food and drinks for everyone, but not much was eaten. We occupied ourselves by telling stories about Tim, many of which included Cryder, and that brought a little light-heartedness to our day.

I had not been with this group of Tim's childhood friends in a long time. I couldn't believe how incredible, mature, loving, and caring they were. They really exposed their hearts, and I can't tell you how close we became in those few hours, how much they helped me get through that day. And the days to come, as well.

Dr. Ruotolo arrived about one and a half hours later to say they had cleaned out the wound, but had to remove more muscle around his ankle than they'd expected. The damaged artery had caused this tissue to die. Then came the more shocking news, which he delivered with little consideration for how he was saying it or to whom he was speaking.

"Tim will probably never be able to lift his toes," he said, "which means he'll need a brace to walk."

I heard Gina gasp at about the same time that I wanted to scream at him for being so insensitive.

"Forever?" I asked.

"Yes."

For the umpteenth time that day my eyes welled up with tears. He went on to say that Tim had handled the surgery well, and they were trying to remove the respirator tube now. When he left, Gina and I hugged and cried again, and then with a stern voice I said to everyone gathered, "No one tell Tim about the brace. I'm not going to accept that; he will be okay."

The room grew silent. I simply was not going to let this happen. I knew Tim, and felt certain he would walk again, without a brace. *I know he will*, I said to myself, just as I'd told myself over and over during the many years of running: *Yes, I will*; and, *Yes, I can*. And, *No, this won't beat me. I won't let it.*

It seemed like a long time before Tim came out of the OR and was being wheeled back to the ICU. I was terrified when I saw him. He was flat on his back. draped in white blankets and sheets with eyes closed. He was white as a ghost and shaking uncontrollably, supposedly "just cold from the OR."

"Please put more blankets on him," I pleaded. "Tim, we're here, we're here. We love you." And Gina was on the other side, stroking his arm and talking to him, too. The tube was out, but he looked awful. At the ICU, all of Tim and Gina's friends stood arm in arm, tears rolling down their cheeks. We all hugged and cried softly together as they wheeled Tim back through the double doors to his curtained spot in the ICU.

One of the surgeons suddenly appeared through the double doors and asked Gina for her help, explaining that Tim needed to stay awake and that they were counting on her voice to do that. Tim's oxygen level had to remain above ninety percent or they would have to reinsert the tube. Tim was having trouble breathing and he could only keep his eyes open for about a minute at a time, if that. Gina was gone for a good five minutes before she appeared in the hallway outside the ICU, calling me in to help keep Tim awake with her. Together we stood by Tim's bed, stroking his arm, hoping that he would sense we were there. We took turns calling his name and could see he was trying hard to open his eyes and pick up his big shaggy head, but just couldn't.

We thought it might help to hear other voices too; it might startle him enough to get him to open his eyes. I was in awe of how all Tim's friends surrounded him, taking turns, trying to keep him breathing. My godson Alex—or, as Tim calls him, his "Godbrother"—stood by the foot of Tim's bed. He was visibly shaken by the whole thing, a look of shock and fear in his eyes.

Tim was not hearing Alex's voice. So I went to the waiting room to get Dave, who had a loud distinctive voice and was the guy with the most outrageous, hysterical stories. But he was more serious than I had ever seen him. Tim was his buddy, and he was there to save him. He clapped his hands and yelled, "Tim, wake up!" Tim's eyes suddenly strained open. It worked! But soon his eyelids closed again and he drifted back into his trance.

The rest of that afternoon and into the night we spent trying to keep Tim awake and breathing. For three hours, every two to four minutes we took turns calling his name. Once in a while my mind would shift to Baltimore and I thought about Lee and wondered how he was doing as he took his first steps. Earlier, I'd had a chance to let him know about Tim's second surgery and he'd told me that of course I needed to stay with our son. He wouldn't dream of having me leave his side.

"Come on Tim, open your eyes . . . open those beautiful blue eyes."

His oxygen level kept drifting down to eighty-eight, eighty-six, eighty-four, and we would yell again. Finally we got him to stay at ninety-four and ninety-five. He began to open his eyes a little more and seemed to be trying to focus on us. Then, miraculously, he opened his eyes wider and looked right at me. Those gorgeous blue eyes were focused right at me. Relief washed through me as I leaned in closer.

"Hi Tim, it's me, Mom . . . you can talk now, the tube is gone. We're here. I love you. Can you say, 'Hi, Mom'?"

And with a very soft whisper, I heard, "Hi, Mom."

"We love you Tim. Can you say 'I love you, Gina'?"

Again, faintly, he managed, "Love you, Gina."

Gina could barely speak as she whispered, "I love you too, Tim." Gina had been through so much, and now Tim was fighting his way back to her, to all of us.

Tim's responsiveness was improving, he was stabilizing. He was starting to ask for food. "Please, cookie? Candy? Pickles?" Tim was coming back. Then he said, "Southside," referring to a specialty drink made with vodka and lemonade. We all started laughing, including my sister Edie, who'd driven down from Rhode Island to lend her support. She and I exchanged a look. There was hope again.

A while later, the attending doctor came by to check his vitals and asked Tim to wiggle his toes on his right foot. They wiggled. Then his left . . . nothing.

"Come on Tim," I begged and touched his left leg to help him realize which toes he was meant to wiggle, thinking he might be too foggy to understand. "Wiggle these toes, Tim, come on you can do it," I begged again. Then, a slight lift of his toes! They moved, up and down! My eyes filled with tears again, "Tim, you moved your toes!"

23

A Bumpy Road and a Smooth One

The next morning (Wednesday), I pulled my one set of clothes out of the dryer and once again put them on. When Edie, Mom, Gina, and I rode up in the hospital elevator with some of Tim's doctors and nurses, I saw them giving us a questioning look. Gina picked up on it and whispered to me, "In case they didn't recognize us, we thought we'd wear the same clothes again for the third day!" We burst into laughter and it felt good to laugh for just a moment.

But my smile faded and a shiver went down my spine as we approached Tim's bed. I sensed the others stiffening as well, and we all pasted on smiles, leaning in to kiss Tim.

He looked very confused as his eyes opened. The oxygen mask cinched tight on his face kept him from talking, but those blue eyes looked at us pleadingly, trying to make sense of what was happening. Gina hid her teary eyes from Tim as she bravely went to work, taking towels to wipe the sweat from his forehead and chest, telling him it was okay, he was doing just fine.

My panic was on the rise again, and so I went in search of his doctors, looking for answers. We all wanted to know why he was sweating so badly. What was wrong? I found his doctor who said he'd made it through the night okay with the oxygen mask, but breathing was still difficult and as a result he was floating in and out of consciousness. But the doctor felt confident he was improving, and this relieved all of us. At least a little.

Lee and I were grateful for all that the ER docs at Nassau University Medical Center, but we agreed that the time had come to have Tim transferred to New York City, where he could see one of the best orthopedic surgeons in the area. I'd decided that I would not leave the hospital that day until I'd managed to arrange the transfer. McNicey back at work!

Past experience had taught me that it was better to speak to someone in person. I went up and down to different floors and administration offices, but it was not proving easy to transfer an ICU patient *and* I was running out of time. I had to catch a train back to Baltimore by early afternoon so I could pick up Lee at Hopkins, as he was going to be discharged. Fortunately, after about an hour and half, I had tracked down everyone I needed to speak with. Mission accomplished!

However, I was terrified of leaving Tim as his condition seemed so precarious, and so I could barely bring myself to say good-bye.

"Be strong," I told him, failing to hold back the tears. "I'll be back in a few days. Gina will take care of you. I love you so much. Don't you stop fighting."

Tim's voice was weak, but he understood I was leaving. "Don't cry, Mom. Please don't."

But I couldn't stop. I gave Tim one last kiss on the cheek and with an aching heart, I hugged Gina and thanked her for watching over Tim, for loving him so much. Of course, she was fighting back tears too and could only hug me. No words were needed.

For most of the train ride back to Baltimore, I was in a trance, staring out the window. For the first time in a while my thoughts turned to Cryder. His senior dinner and final game were this weekend, only three days away. Would Lee be strong enough to go? Would Tim be okay? How *was* Lee doing? So many thoughts cycled through my mind, and again and again I tried to stay focused on the here and now, on what we needed to do next, just as I always had when preparing for a race, or competing in a triathlon. One stroke at a time, one push of the pedal, one step. And, somehow, you finish the race.

I found my car where I had left it a couple of days earlier and drove to the other side of Hopkins, then went inside to pick Lee up in the main building. I could hardly believe I was about to see him—my skinny, bald husband. Then, there he was, with the biggest smile and arms ready to embrace me as I peeked around the corner. Being held by him gave me the comfort I had been yearning for.

He was still in his hospital nightie, which made me laugh. "You can't go home in that!" Of course I had come straight from the train and had no other clothes for him, so he would have to ear the nightie. He wore a full-length leg brace, aimed at keeping him from bending his leg and irritating the stitches, but which also prevented him from getting his pants on. I tried not to think of Tim in such a brace.

We were home by five thirty and so happy to be there. The following morning the phone rang at six and my heart skipped a beat when I heard Tim's voice. He almost sounded normal again. He had been moved to New York City during the night and was in his new room, though as always seemed to be the case with Tim, there was a story to be told.

Apparently, Tim had woken up the night before and was confused as to why he was still in the ICU. He somehow got hold of a phone and called his uncle John. Tim knew John had been helping us with his transfer to Hospital for Special Surgery. Problem was, it was two in the morning. John said that after his heart stopped racing on hearing the phone ring, he picked up the receiver and heard, "Uncle John?"

"Yes, Tim?"

"Uncle John, I'm still here in the ICU."

John chuckled. "Tim, it's two in the morning. I'll see what I can do first thing after I get up." And, of course, in due time Tim was transferred.

When I spoke to the orthopedic surgeon's nurse, she assured me that Tim was being well cared for and that nothing further would be done on his leg until the following week. He would not be ready for another surgery until then, so it looked like we'd be safe to travel to Chapel

Hill for Cryder's game and celebration dinner, assuming Lee felt strong enough to go. Before we made the final decision, though, we called Tim who absolutely insisted we go. We then called Cryder, who said he completely understood if we could not be there, that it was far more important we be with Tim and he would have some of our friends stand in for us. But, after receiving Tim's blessing, wild horses were not going to keep Lee from standing on that lacrosse field with Cryder.

I did worry about the huge incision in the back of Lee's leg, which stretched from the middle of his butt all the way down to just above the back of his knee, with a drain that emptied into a plastic container, and which Nurse McNicey had to empty each time it filled. If he was in pain, though, he was keeping it to himself, and he was getting around amazingly well.

Senior Day was something we'd been planning for months, for years even. It was a big tribute to Cryder and all the seniors on the team, the culmination of their years of dedication and hard work. It would also be bittersweet—the end of Cryder's years of playing lacrosse for UNC. That would leave a hole in our lives, for sure, but we couldn't wait to celebrate his career, a once in a lifetime event. A celebration, in fact, would be a nice change.

I was up early on Friday morning, and had everything all packed up and ready to go by ten a.m., when we got a phone call from Dr. Attar's nurse at Hopkins. Lee's expression darkened and his whole body seemed to deflate; I could tell she'd delivered some bad news.

I was almost afraid to ask. "What's wrong?" I said timidly.

"She said Dr. Attar would not like me traveling by car and moving around so much. We should stay home." I sat in stunned silence for a couple of minutes. Then a solution occurred to me. McNicey to the rescue.

"What if I make a bed in the back of the car so you can lie back and keep your leg up? What would be the difference between reclining in a car and sitting on a sofa?"

"How would you do that?" Lee asked hopefully.

"Well, I am a very resourceful person!" I found some foam pool floats, cushions, and pillows and made a perfect size bed in the back of

Cryder's SUV, which he had swapped for my car when he'd driven up a few days earlier, thinking we might need the bigger car to transport Lee. And he'd been right.

Lee came out to inspect it and a big smile came across his face. "Leave it to McNicey!"

"Climb on in. Let's go!"

I have to admit that I was really nervous about driving Lee to Chapel Hill. If anything happened, I'd feel terribly guilty. My one comfort was that I knew my good friend Lauren would be there, and she's a critical care nurse. Of course, there was always the UNC medical center, too. Still, a little nagging voice in my head kept saying, *Be careful!*

Driving through DC was a bit congested with bumps and turns. At one point, as I heard him rolling towards the right, he called out, "Hey, remember I'm back here!" Of course I knew he was back there, I put him there!

Cryder's smile spread across his face as Lee hobbled over on his crutches to greet him. Luckily, Cryder had thought ahead and asked if the trainers would transport Lee from the parking lot to the field in one of the golf carts for the game—another problem solved. It would be challenge enough for Lee to get across the field. The Carolina family was in awe of Lee making it to the game on Saturday only five days after surgery. Everyone wanted to hug him, and he loved it!

Game day was a gorgeous day. The senior parents all lined up on the sideline before thegame and as each senior was honored, the parents would meet their son in the middle of the field for a photo. When it was our turn, we started a little early before they introduced us to give Lee a head start on his crutches while I walked with him. The announcers were reeling off Cryder's accomplishments and stats, but I heard nothing. I was mesmerized by the whole scene, watching Cryder jog to meet us with a smile that would light up the world. I could hear Lee swallowing hard and glanced at him to see his eyes brimming with tears.

Cryder carried a bouquet of flowers, which he forgot to hand to me, instead choosing to hug his Dad first, then me. I could see in

Cryder's eyes that he was holding back tears, too. The Carolina family was hollering and cheering, not only for Cryder but also for Lee. I, too, was swallowing hard, trying to suppress the wave of emotion rolling across the field. It was a moment I'm sure the three of us will never forget, followed by the game, against Ohio State, a close one, with the win making the celebration that night all the better.

All the speeches made to the sons during Senior Dinner were incredibly touching. When Lee started his speech, Cryder, who sat between us, focused on the plate in front of him. I know he was afraid to look at his father and see him struggle with the emotion of telling his son how proud he was of him. In fact, I think our whole table might have been staring at their plates! In the end, there were lots of hugs with all the parents and all the boys. A tight family for four years, we were now saying good-bye.

Later, after it was all over, Cryder walked us out to the car, stopping at his own car and reappearing with two bouquets of flowers and two Mother's Day cards, one from him and one from Tim. I was speechless. This time I couldn't hold back my tears. I was so caught off guard, completely forgetting one of my favorite Hallmark events! It was an incredibly thoughtful gesture and I felt so loved. I reveled in the moment until I thought of Tim and remembered how long of a way we had to go until the four of us were once more together, relaxing and joking and having a Southside.

24

The Next Steps

Before falling into bed Sunday night, I had to repack for our trip up to New York. We were both anxious to be with Tim, particularly Lee who had not seen Tim since before his accident. From all our phone conversations, Tim was doing well, in large part because Gina was managing the flow of visitors so Tim could get much-needed rest. An amazing young woman, she was juggling work, hospital visits of friends and family, and trying to find some time to see Tim alone. With her apartment located at the other end of the city, her task was all the more daunting. I worried about her, too, and we hoped to relieve her of some of her "McNicey" duties when we got to the city.

Before heading up to New York on Monday morning we had to stop at Hopkins for Lee's first checkup since the surgery. It was amazing that a week had passed since Lee's tumor had been removed. He already looked healthier and stronger. We weren't sure if any reports would be back yet. I, for one, refused to think anything but positive thoughts, although my breath always did catch a little when the doors opened to the examining room and the doctor walked in.

Is he smiling? Is he looking concerned? Please, no bad news. That morning, Dr. Attar was all smiles. He could not wait to share the best news of all. The pathology report had come back. The margins around the tumor were clean! And the tumor itself, which they tested after removing it, had shown little signs of life. In other words, the chemo and the radiation treatments had pretty much killed it! It was one of the best days ever.

We found our way to the information desk at the NewYork-Presbyterian/Weill Cornell Medical Center, where Tim had to remain because he needed to be in a hospital with an ICU unit, and Hospital for Special Surgery didn't have one. But the two hospitals were attached by a skywalk. It is a huge complex and it was a long walk to Tim's room. Lee was trying to weave his way through the crowds behind me while I tried to make a path for him.

Finally, we found Tim and a big smile spread across his face as our eyes met. Lee hobbled in on his crutches behind me and over to Tim's bed. The two of them hugged and hugged. What a beautiful sight. When Lee pulled away, tears were running down his cheeks, and Tim's eyes were brimming, too.

Lee was clearly shocked to see the extent of Tim's injuries. Tim's leg was being held in place by an external fixator, a big metal cage around his leg, with two long screws into his shin bone. It is very heavy and, needless to say, makes him a prisoner in bed. You could see the wound, and it was gruesome. There was a eight by three -inch swath without any muscle or tissue from about mid-shin down to his ankle. A black sponge-like bandage covered the wound and was sealed by a clear bandage, making the wound very visible. Large stitches closed up long gashes in several places on his legs. Luckily, Lee couldn't see the back of his own leg. I think he would have been pretty horrified by that, too. Of course, Tim tried to make light of his wounds, saying he thought he might have outdone his father. Wonderful!

Gina soon appeared around the doorway and the very happy reunion was complete. Gina's strength and love for Tim had been unfaltering. I owed her so much for being there for Tim when I could not.

We had made it a priority to meet Dr. Helfet. We wanted to know exactly what was involved in repairing Tim's injuries. Could they be fixed? Would Tim walk again? Would he wear a brace for the rest of his life? Would he be in a wheelchair? How long did the doctor expect Tim to be in the hospital? What would his recovery time be? So many unknowns. And then there was also the fact that I would be needed in Baltimore to take care of Lee. We weren't planning to move to New York. How could I manage caring for them both?

When we'd spoken to Gina, out of earshot of Tim, we told her this was a lot for her to deal with and we didn't expect her to take care of Tim. That was our job. She looked at us with this bewildered expression and said, "Oh, Mr. and Mrs. D, I want to take care of Tim. I wouldn't be anywhere else. This is not a burden for me." That said it all. Tim was a lucky man and we were so grateful.

I found my way over to Dr. Helfet's office. It was a long walk, so Lee stayed with Tim. We sat in his office and he told me with total certainty that Tim would walk again and without a brace. Words I was dying to hear, but still the relief I felt was so unexpected and happy tears stung my eyes. However, he couldn't deny that Tim would have a long road ahead of him after his next major surgery—scheduled for the following week—when a rod would be inserted in his leg and muscle and tissue transplanted from his abdomen to cover the bone, followed by a skin graft to cover the tissue.

He was very complimentary about Tim, saying how well he was handling the trauma and he believed Tim was up to the challenge. Tim would be in a wheelchair for a while and then on crutches. We discussed rehab. I told him Tim wanted to stay in New York and go back to his apartment and have his girlfriend take care of him. He frowned and said, "I would advise against that. Nine times out of ten, the boyfriend or girlfriend is out the door in a week when they are faced with a situation like Tim's."

"I can see how that might be true," I said, "but I really don't think Gina would do that. They have been together for six years, and she has been amazing with him. She said she wants to take care of him."

He nodded skeptically. Whether Tim would need to be in a rehab facility or could return to his apartment from the hospital would depend on how he made it through the big surgery and how well he recovered. It would be difficult for him to maneuver a wheelchair and a walker in his tiny apartment in New York. But we needed to take things one day at a time. First, we had to get Tim through his major surgery the following week. After our meeting, I had great confidence in Dr. Helfet. Trauma cases like Tim's were his specialty, and I liked his assuredness.

I received a touching email from Tim's friend Max, the one who'd called us about Tim's accident eleven days after the event:

Hey, Mrs. D,

I just wanted to write to say how incredibly sorry I am about Tim's accident, and to say congratulations on Mr. D's successful surgery; he looks great! I know it has been a lot to process in a short amount of time, but your two guys are the toughest I've met and I am continually impressed with Tim's fortitude and strength throughout his recovery, as I am sure everyone has been with Mr. D's as well. Tim has a great support group of friends who love him a lot, me included, who will be there for him through the whole process. Happy belated Mother's Day, and so happy you liked the flowers. Lots of love to you and the whole fam, and please don't hesitate to write or call if there is anything at all Sarah or I can do to help out. Otherwise we will be in to visit Tim on Monday and give him his first tutorial on his iPad, although I am sure he will figure it all out well before then.

Max

I wrote back to Max the next day:

That is the sweetest email. I know you feel horribly responsible for Tim because it happened at your house and on your "toy." But it was not your fault and I do not throw any blame at all in your direction. You have been a very, very special friend to Tim and, trust me, I know you would never do anything to hurt him. I always worry about Tim, because many times he leaps before he thinks, especially when he's with the boys! I have always loved Tim's sense of adventure, but he does need a little voice in his ear saying, sure you want to do that?!

Tim has told me many times how amazing you and Sarah have been for both him and Gina through this whole ordeal. I experienced that myself with those few days we all spent in Nassau County Medical Center together. Through all my tears, I could see in both your and Sarah's eyes the love and concern you have for Tim. It was a rough time, but one that made a lot of us think about how precious life and friends are. I want to thank you for all you've done for Tim. I know you spearheaded the iPad gift idea. Wow, what an incredibly generous, thoughtful gift. It will most definitely help occupy his time. Thanks, Max, for your incredibly sweet email and for all you've done for Tim.

With love, Mrs. D

25

The Final Push

That spring, I spent endless hours driving up and down the highway between New York and Baltimore. If I had to be in a car, I'd much prefer to be the passenger and while away a long drive leafing through magazines. I hate sitting still! But, with Lee's condition, I was the sole driver, and my poor car was accumulating mileage like mad.

On Monday, May 17, I sent out an email updating people of Tim's and Lee's status:

> On Wednesday, Tim had his third "washout" surgery. We got there early morning so we could see Dr. Helfet. While we were sitting in the waiting room, I looked over at Lee and noticed some very light, soft whiskers coming in on his lip and chin!!!! His hair was growing back! So exciting! Nothing on his head yet . . . keep referring to him as my Chia Pet . . . waiting for the sprouts to show. Also another big step forward for Lee . . . on Thursday he had the drain removed from his leg!! I had to clean that drain and empty the plastic bottle of fluid two times a day. Most of my nursing care has been very manageable, but this job was not my favorite and most certainly has helped me conclude that I do not want to be McNicey forever!!

So back to Tim . . . Dr. H said there was no more sign of infection!!! The plan is to do one more washout surgery (which they did on Saturday) and then the big surgery on Tuesday (tomorrow).

Just to keep you updated on lacrosse: on Saturday morning Lee and I went down to Chapel Hill for the first game of the NCAA playoffs. UNC played Delaware last night in a nail biter. They won 13-12 after an hour and a half rain delay. I will let you all know how Tim's surgery goes, but want to let you know that my #1 patient is amazing and getting stronger every second. Soon he will be out on the golf course again with a big smile on his face and hopefully some hair on his head! As for Tim, please keep the prayers going . . . he has a tough couple of months ahead and this surgery is going to be a long one. Thanks to all of you. lots of love.

Xox

On Monday, the day before Tim's big surgery, Lee and I climbed into the car once again to head north to New York, arriving in the late afternoon at Tim's hospital bed. I was amazed at how much Tim had improved since we last saw him. His beard was getting longer, and he looked incredibly handsome! He was in good spirits and anxious to have the big surgery done first thing in the morning. He had been stuck in the same position in bed for seventeen days, with that big cage screwed into his leg. I don't know how he did it. He never complained about anything. He was so thankful. This time, we only stayed a little while. Everyone was tired, and the following day was going to be a long one.

I woke early Tuesday morning after a sleepless night worrying about Tim's big day. I threw on my running gear and snuck out the door, dashing down First Avenue to arrive at the hospital by six a.m. I had agreed to meet Gina there so we could see Tim for one more hug before he was wheeled off to surgery. Tim shook his head and smiled when I arrived in his room wearing running clothes, as I explained it was much quicker than waiting for a cab!

The plastic surgeon team stopped in and explained that they would take the muscle from his side to fill in the missing tissue and muscle by his tibia. They would take the skin from his "good" thigh for the graft. My poor boy was going to be a mass of scars. He did ask that maybe they could try to keep the graft and scar on his side hidden so he would still look (really) good in his bathing suits! I had to laugh as there were so many scars all over his body already but I loved the fact that Tim was concerned about his bathing suit line. While we were waiting for Tim to be wheeled out he told me he finally saw the X-ray of the busted tibia and said it looked like someone had taken a baseball bat to his shin. I was just totally shattered. Well, Tim never likes to do things halfway!

They finally came to wheel Tim to the OR around seven thirty. . We wished him luck with a group hug and promised we would be waiting for him when he was done. Next time I would see him he would finally have the horrible external fixator off and be able to move his leg after two weeks of one position in bed. A huge step forward and such a relief for Tim.

It was a long day as we all gathered in the waiting room. My mother came in from Long Island to keep Gina, Lee, and me company.

After a few hours of sitting in the stiff vinyl upholstered chairs, Lee turned to me and whispered, "Is this what we are going to do all day? Do we just sit here?"

I had to chuckle a little because I had become so accustomed to "just sitting" in hospitals, but now the shoe was on the other foot for Lee. This time he was not the patient!

Another hour went by and Dr. Helfet came out of surgery to find us in the waiting room. He told us he was thrilled with the way the surgery was going. He was able to straighten the bones and place the plate over the fracture. All was secure and looked really good with plenty of blood supply. Wow! We were so relieved! The next part of the surgery was the long part and he promised to check back in with us around one thirty. The waiting seemed endless as we tried to amuse ourselves with books, magazines, Tim's iPad, or just idle chatter.

Finally around two o'clock, Dr. Helfet came back into the waiting room and explained that Dr. Gael (the head plastic surgeon) was removing the muscle flap from Tim's abdomen and was going to place it over the plate. Tim was doing really well and Dr. Gael would be out to see us around three thirty. Dr. Helfet said he also had to do a bone graft, which he luckily got from the bone bank, so no new scar for that!

By four o'clock I was really beginning to feel antsy. Tim had been under anesthesia since eight that morning, and I was getting worried. I found myself pacing more and more and watching the door to the waiting room, willing some news from our doctors. Finally the nurse rotating through the OR to bring news back to waiting families reported that Tim was doing fine, the flap was in place, and they were connecting the vessels, etc. This, she emphasized, was the intricate part, and they probably wouldn't be done until around six thirty. Wow! We were expecting a five- to six-hour surgery, not nine hours.

Finally, around six fifteen, Dr. Gael walked in the room. I had never met Dr. Gael before but by now we were the last family in the waiting room so he didn't have to ask at the nurse desk which family was Tim's. He greeted us with a warm smile and happily told us the surgery was a success. He was able to transplant the muscle to the tibia where all the muscle and tendons were missing. He explained how he went up through his abdomen (keeping the incision under his bathing suit line, so no visible tummy scar for Tim!), took three of his "six pack," and spliced it onto the muscle at his ankle and below his knee. That muscle would act as a conductor between the two muscles and allow the foot to dorsiflex, so he could walk. He was also able to repair the nerve. Amazing! I don't know how those doctors do what they do while standing on their feet for hours and hours focusing on such intricate work.

He went on to say it would probably take about six months for the muscle to fully connect and allow the foot to properly respond. Tim would have to wear a brace to help him walk for the next six months, but hopefully after that, he'd be OK. He would not have as much range as he did before, but he was going to walk! Suddenly I could breath again. My boy was going to be OK. The doctor's words were what I was yearning to hear. I couldn't help but hug him and tell him how grateful we were.

We were allowed into recovery around six forty-five. Lee and I went first and as I rounded the corner to Tim's curtained stall, I was not sure what we would find. I rubbed his arm and softly called his name. His eyes opened immediately and a slight smile spread across his lips. He looked amazingly well for nine hours of surgery, but was obviously in pain and pretty beat up. Still, he was very aware of what was going on. I excitedly told him the surgery was a success and that he would walk again, and as my words sunk in, Tim's eyes filled and brimmed over. I wiped away the tears and hugged him tight. Happy news, for a change!

We left soon after to allow Gina her turn with Tim and promised to be back first thing in the morning. We were told Tim would be in the ICU for the next two days so they could carefully monitor the flap and skin graft and make sure that no clots formed where they transplanted muscle. If that were to happen, it would mean they would have to go back in and start all over. I didn't even want to think about that, and thankfully Doctor Gael said there was a less than five percent chance of that happening. I was comforted to know he would be monitored carefully!

Lee and I could barely drag ourselves back to the apartment and fell into bed. I woke several times worried about Tim and hoping he was not in too much pain. In the morning, while Lee was still sleeping. I snuck out the door for my favorite loop in Central Park. The sun was rising and it was going to be a good day!

It's Saturday morning and tomorrow will be three weeks since Tim's accident and almost three weeks since Lee's surgery. On Wednesday, I gave Lee the last injections! McNicey is winding down!! He still has a little trouble bending down to put his pants on (so he claims!!) so I do have to help him, but we are DILIGENTLY working on that flexibility! He even went to work on Thursday and Friday for full days of work. (A little free time for me!!! Hooray!) I am still the chauffeur, but he is really hoping that will change soon . . . me too!

Apparently Lee's surgery was watched by many doctors because it was one of the biggest sarcomas they've ever seen! Lee did sign a video release before surgery and is now concerned his derriere will be featured on YouTube!

Back to Tim. On Wednesday morning, Tim was still in the ICU and in a lot of pain, mostly his abdomen where they removed the muscle, but he was in good spirits and able to move his left leg without the cage on it anymore. While we were there, Dr. Helfet's nurse touched his left foot, checking for "feeling" and asking if he could move his toes. He couldn't move his big toe yet, but his foot and leg were very swollen from the surgery and hopefully that feeling will all come back soon. They had a monitor on his foot to check the pulse to make sure there was continual blood flow.

By Thursday morning, he sounded like a new person. The doctors had been in to do their rounds and told him all looked very good. Brewster (his incredibly devoted uncle, who has been to visit Tim almost every other day . . . so grateful to him!!) stopped by again and reported that Tim's color was much better and he seemed pretty good. Tim also got a surprise visit from his best Aunt EVER . . . Edie drove all the way from Newport for the day so she could give him a hug and deliver her famous chocolate chip cookies. Tim was so touched. Thank you, Edie, you are the best!!

Yesterday morning Tim called and was seemingly on cloud nine. He'd had visits from both the plastics and the ortho teams. Plastics said everything looked really good. They are planning on "unveiling" the flap/graft on Sunday. If all looked good, he would be able to start to hang his leg over the bed and begin in-hospital therapy. Since the surgery, he has had to keep his leg elevated so no blood clots settle in his leg. The ortho doc then told him that his right leg is now approved to hold one hundred percent of his weight!!! That means he'll be able to use a walker and/or crutches and not be restricted to a wheelchair.

Must be our family genes . . . good bones and fast healers!! There is, of course, the power of positive thinking and all the love and prayers sent by all of you. This morning I woke to an email from Tim that he was moved out of the ICU last night at 11 p.m. and is now on the eighth floor. Most of his monitors and lines have been removed. Progress!!!

We are leaving in an hour to head up to Princeton to watch Cryder's game. UNC plays Duke in the second round of the NCAA championship today at two thirty. Can you all please send those powerful positive vibes you've been sending to the UNC lacrosse team . . . we need extra help on this one . . . Duke has been on fire and we are not ready for Cryder's career in lacrosse to end just yet. Hoping they make it one more round! We miss Tim's spirit on the sidelines!! Hope you all have a great weekend. Love to everyone.

xoxox

Sadly, the Duke game didn't end in our favor, though our boys played a great first half. And so ended Cryder's awesome lacrosse career. It was a time we cherished, and we felt fortunate that Cryder lived his dream, playing for UNC. When the game ended and the team shook hands, we watched with heavy hearts.

As Cryder walked off the field, he turned back to the stands and raised his arm to wave to us. My throat closed up and my eyes began to sting. I was so proud of him. The postgame tailgate wasn't as high energy as they had been for most of the season. It was a tough moment to swallow, watching all those senior boys shake hands with the parents who had supported them for the last four years. I wish we could have taken Cryder with us for the night and then on to New York the next morning. I knew he was anxious to see Tim. But that was not how it worked; the team traveled back home together. As the boys climbed onto the bus and waved good-bye, my heart was aching and I felt hollow. It was over. All those years cheering in the stands had come to an end.

Later on Saturday, Lee and I said our good-byes to everyone in our UNC family—a bittersweet moment—and headed to our hotel. We called Tim along the way. Just hearing his voice lifted our spirits.

"Hi, Mom! Guess who's sitting in a chair?"

"What? Are you kidding?" I couldn't believe it. He said they had moved him onto a "high" chair that they brought into his room and placed by his bed. The nurses moved him onto the chair while they kept his leg out straight and placed it on the bed. It was the first time he had been off his back in three weeks. He was ecstatic! We were going to celebrate that night after all, so we'd drink a toast to Tim's health and Cryder's career, too.

The next morning, Sunday, we drove like madmen, desperate to get back to Tim. It was going to be a difficult day for Tim and we needed to be there. He was supposed to have his bandage removed from his graft (the unveiling) and start his first therapy. We arrived in time and the therapists began to remove the bandage. I was prepared to be a bit shocked because Dr. Gael had described what it would look like, but, wholly moly, it looked like an alien head coming out of his leg and I had to work hard not to let Tim see my horrified reaction.

The next step for Tim was to swing his legs over the bed and let his legs dangle over the edge for five minutes. Sounded easy enough, but it had been three weeks since Tim's legs had been bent and low-ered. He was so excited for this moment. Brewster was there as well and we both had our cell phones ready to snap photos, in fact Brew was going to videotape it. As Tim swung around in bed, two physical therapists helped him maneuver and then began to slowly lower Tim's left leg over the side of the bed. They had not yet finished when Tim began to scream with pain and we instantly turned our cameras off.

The therapists controlled the lowering of his leg and Tim's screams turned to heavy breathing and groans of pain.

I'm not sure if it was Tim's pain or the wound or the fact that Lee was standing next to the eighth floor window (he doesn't like heights), but suddenly Lee felt nauseous and had to leave the room. Tim's face turned very white and you could see he was struggling. Tim thought it was going to be such a simple move just to hang his legs over the edge of the bed for five minutes, but it was so much harder and obviously so much more painful than he'd anticipated.

All the while, I was sending him my thoughts—*Manage the pain, Tim, breathe, rise above it*—and recalled ever so briefly the race in which I catapulted over the handlebars of my bike coming into the transition area at the end of the bike portion of the Oyster Bay Triathlon. I managed to pick myself up, rack my bike, and continue onto the 5k run portion. The pain was searing through my shoulder, but I refused to let the pain stop me, and, with my thumb hooked into my speedo bathing suit strap to keep my arm from jiggling, I finished in first place for the women. Right after the race they took me to the hospital where I was told I broke my collarbone. The doctors insisted on surgery right away as it was a compound fracture and the bone had pierced through the skin behind my shoulder. "How did you run like that?" they asked, appearing quite surprised. I'd shut the pain out, compartmentalized it, I told them, and that's what I was hoping Tim would learn to do now.

In that moment Tim realized this was going to be a longer haul than he'd expected. Slowly, they raised his leg, turning Tim and placing his legs back on the bed. The physical therapists then checked the wound again to make sure it had handled the extra blood flow and that all looked good. The physical therapists' plan was to increase the leg dangle by five minutes every day until he reached thirty minutes. At twenty minutes, they would have him try to stand for the first time. When all this was achieved, he would be released to go home. We stayed with Tim for a while after that first day, but that little bit of exertion had wiped him out. So we left and let him sleep.

Since Tim was a bit discouraged from the first attempt, two hours prior to the next session he raised the back of his bed making himself sit up in bed, getting his body used to being upright after spending so much time lying flat on his back. The afternoon therapy proved just as difficult, and again he was wiped out.

All the times we spent sitting with Tim we talked about many things. He'd had a lot of time to think about all that had happened in his life. Tim was not entirely a different person, but he had changed in the three weeks since the accident.

In one of our quiet moments during that visit, he wanted to talk to me about his friend David who had been driving the Gator when the accident happened. David had stopped by a few times to see Tim at the hospital in New York, and he'd told Tim how sorry he was, but Tim knew I was having a hard time facing David, in large part because David had never called us to apologize or reached out in any way. He wanted me to bury the hatchet and reach out to him. He was worried about the problems David was having because of the accident—not really physical problems because, as often seems to happen, the driver was able to walk away.

The time we'd unexpectedly seen David occurred on the evening Lee saw Tim in the hospital for the first time. Lee, Gina, and I had been with Tim for about an hour when David walked in, limping a little and with a cane. He and Tim had been friends in grade school, so I hadn't seen him in years, but I recognized him instantly. Lee did not.

As David walked into the hospital room, I felt my body stiffen. I politely greeted him, and then Lee shook his hand, asking him, also politely, what had happened to him?

"Oh," he said, with a pathetic look and feeble voice, "I was the unfortunate driver." I watched Lee's surprised reaction and felt my grip tighten on Tim's bedside railings. For the next ten minutes or so, David told us about how he had come from physical therapy because his legs, which had been bruised in the accident, bothered him when he sat or climbed the stairs. It took everything I had not to grab him and shake him. I think we were all stunned as we sat and listened. I am sure it was a difficult meeting for him, too, and maybe he was just nervous and didn't know what to say. But "Mr. and Mrs. DiPietro, I am so incredibly sorry for this accident" would have been a better way to start.

The next morning when I went for my run in Central Park, I started thinking about the meeting with David and all that he'd said and hadn't said. I started running faster and faster as I grew angrier and angrier. During that run, I composed a letter in my head to David, telling him how I felt. I would not be able to face him again if I didn't speak my mind. When I got back from my run, I wrote that private note, making it clear to David that I did not blame him for the accident itself. Accidents happen, and I did feel terrible for him that he was the driver. But what infuriated me was his audacity to stand at the foot of Tim's bed, in front of Tim's broken body, and complain about his bruises without so much as an apology to us.

It had now been more than three weeks since Tim's accident, however, and two weeks since I had written that first note without a response from David. I knew from what Tim had told me that something was haunting David terribly. After all, he was a good friend of Tim's—it had to be haunting him. But Tim was right. I had to move on, too. First, though, there was another note I needed to write to David, and I copied Tim so he would know what I said and learn from the message as well.

David,

I spoke with Tim last night and he asked me to reach out to you because he is very worried about YOU. Leave it to Tim to always be thinking about someone else's situation. I have to say that one of Tim's most wonderful attributes is his compassion and concern for others. He said he has had many talks with you and is very concerned about how difficult this whole accident has been for you. That he would hate to be in your shoes, and have to face Tim every day, blaming yourself for this accident. I agree; a very difficult place to be. As I said to you before, I hold Tim as responsible for the accident as you. I am quite sure that you were both egging each other on. I also am very aware of Tim's "thrill seeking" nature and his, sometimes, fly-by-the-seat-of-his-pants decisions. It has scared me for years. I always worried when he was with "the boys" without a level-headed woman or friend to curb his behavior. I think all you guys encouraged a little bit of wild behavior, with very little thought to consequences. Being responsible for your actions, and understanding the effects they have, not only on you, but on people that love and care for you, comes with maturity.

One thing I have always said to my boys is there is always something good that comes out of something bad. It is up to you to find that "good" and hold onto that and move forward. It doesn't do you any good to dwell on what has happened . . . you can't change that, and feeling sorry for yourself is not going to make it better either. I know Tim has spent a lot of time thinking about what has happened and how it will change his life for the better. He now understands that many of the risks he has taken in the past were irresponsible and could have led to some truly disastrous outcomes. He is hopeful that this accident has not only opened his eyes and changed his life, but that his friends will benefit from this horrible accident and realize that it's time to be more thoughtful about choices and risks that you take.

David, I know this has been tough on you. But it is up to you to turn it into a positive and use this accident to share with others and help them make better decisions. You should try to find a professional to talk to and help you get through this. It helps to talk about it so you can understand your feelings. It does not do any good to hide from it. It happened, and you have to move forward. Tim is a survivor and he will get through this. I am thankful that he has discovered how precious life is and how many people love him.

We, as a family, have come to appreciate that the love and support of our friends and family are a powerful healing tool. Keep your chin up and be positive.

　　Best, Mrs. D

I felt much better after I wrote that note to David. I was freeing myself from the anger and hopefully helping David learn from a terrible accident. It was time to go back to Baltimore, and hopefully the next trip to New York would be to spring Tim from the hospital.

　　Suffice it to say that the road to recovery for Tim was fraught with setbacks, but Tim was persistent, something I think I'll claim a little credit for. Throughout his youth he witnessed the work and endless training I did to get in shape, and he got to see the payoff when he came to watch me run, swim, and bike competitively. From this I think he'd learned a little about muscle strengthening and understood the value of hard work. He also tended to have a great attitude, something I certainly tried to encourage. During his rehab, there were certainly times when I could hear the discouragement in his voice, but he always assured us that he was NOT giving up! And he didn't.

　　Tim went from a leg dangle of five minutes to ten, fifteen, and so on. Then he began to try to sit in a chair, but blacked out after ten minutes. When he was finally ready to stand up for the first time, three and a half weeks after the accident, he was excited but also scared. He stood for thirty seconds and it was very painful and his blood pressure dropped precipitously. A few days later, he walked. His first independent "stroll" happened using a walker; he went from his hospital bed to the bathroom and back. You can't imagine his euphoria, and ours. The very next day, he was ready to leave the hospital.

Tim's eyes closed as the wind hit him, and I could see him take a deep breath.

　　"How does that feel," I asked, having just rolled Tim's wheelchair through the hospital doors.

"Awesome," he said, smiling. It was Tim's first time outside since May 2, one day shy of four weeks. We were heading to Mom and Jack's, where he'd be staying for the first phase of his rehab. When I had mentioned to Mom that I didn't know what to do when Tim was released and where to take him, she volunteered immediately, knowing he wanted to stay close to Gina and close to his doctors. I was so relieved but also not sure if they knew how much work it would be. He'd be in a wheelchair for several weeks, and also using a walker. They would have to clean his wounds, help him bath, lift him on the toilet . . . It was a lot to ask.

When we pulled into Mom and Jack's, Tim had an even bigger smile on his face. Brewster and his kids had decorated the front gate with "Welcome Home" banners and balloons. Mom and Jack, Brew and the kids, and Kitty and George were all waiting for Tim and clapping as we drove in. He was home! We maneuvered him back out of the car and Jack insisted on wheeling him all the way to the front terrace. He hadn't seen Tim since he stood at his bed in the ICU and now was taking him under his care. It was a beautiful, sunny day, and we all sat out and enjoyed lunch with Tim. it was such a great moment.

Just when you think things are settling down, though, you get the one-two punch again. I was worried that Tim's recuperation at my parent's house was going to be a burden, but I never anticipated he would end up back in the emergency room the day after he got there!

Brewster again spent most of the night in the ER with Tim and Gina. He had been by Tim's side many, many hours throughout this whole ordeal. Brewster was more than an uncle to Tim; he was like his big brother, a best friend.

What we thought might be a terrible setback actually turned out to be an episode of kidney stones. Painful, but what an incredible relief. We had been fearful that another surgery might be more than Tim could take.

When he once again returned to my mother's, she and Jack had set up a lounge chair for him on the patio overlooking Oyster Bay Harbor. It was quite a view and one that Tim relished nearly every day of his stay. But I also insisted that my mother and Brewster not wait on him hand and foot. I asked them to make him get up and get a glass of water. The more he used his muscles, the faster they would come back. I knew it was hard to watch him struggle, but it was important to use a little tough love too.

As for Lee, he had abandoned his leg brace, much to Dr. Attar's surprise when we visited in late May.

"No cane or crutches?" Dr. Attar asked.

"Oh, well, um, I don't really feel I need those either," said Lee.

Dr. Attar, with a big smile said, "Well, that's great . . . can't believe it!"

The incision looked fine, and although Lee tried to convince him to take out some of the stitches, Dr. Attar said he was a strong candidate for wound problems because of the radiated skin and the size of the incision, and so he felt that Lee should leave them in for another two weeks. A big step Lee made was driving himself to work . . . no more McNicey the chauffeur! With Lee at the office and working full days, I suddenly had the house to myself again.

And then the doctors discovered that Lee had developed an infection in his stitches and the drain needed to be reinserted. This was another blow for Lee, but luckily it was only a twenty-four-hour stay in the hospital,

A couple of days later, I was most appreciative of an email that my mother's friend had written to her and Mom had forwarded to me:

The good news is that Lee hasn't sent any emails for a while. I can't tell you how hard it has been on her fan club struggling to keep up with the frenetic pace of developments in the DiPietro family . . . most of them terrifying! The fact that we are looking at great results all around, I think is due to Lee's single-minded determination that this is how it must be! I have never seen anyone display such a ferocious will in the face of so much bad news. When Lee told Tim to move his toes and he did, it was clear who was in charge of the situation. And did anyone ever doubt there would be an email (a hilarious, tear-jerking email) describing the discharge from the hospital and the drive to UNC?

The good doctors' meaningless predictions meant nothing with McNicey running the show. Lee would be cured and Tim would walk, period! Honestly, Nina, I have never read anything so hair-raising—like a fast-paced thriller whose author's goal is to keep her readers in a state of permanent terror. And while you are at it, maybe you can explain how Lee managed to write one beautifully detailed update after another in the midst of trying to cope with the crazy logistics of husband and son in parallel trauma so many miles apart. Now, finally, I know what an Iron Woman is.

26

A New Phase

We had our setbacks, but during the week leading up to Father's Day things noticeably began to return to normal as both Lee and Tim gained strength and confidence. I even imagined I might have time to hit a few golf balls with a friend the next time I visited Tim, though I often used my long early-morning runs to process what was happening in my life which took the free time I had, leaving little time for golf. I often thought it would have been great during Lee's and Tim's ordeals if I could have carried a tape recorder, because during the runs I composed my emails and then would go directly to the computer and write it all down when I returned.

Subject: 68 Days post-chemo
Lee had his appointment with Dr. Attar yesterday afternoon. He was somewhat hesitant to go back to Hopkins after last week. We had gotten an email earlier in the day from Dr. Attar's nurse, saying the cultures taken during the surgery had originally come back negative, but had grown something over the weekend. We are expecting a call from the infectious disease docs re: antibiotic treatment. Lee was worried they were going to put in another port for an IV drip.

On our way to the hospital he told me if they try to keep him in Hopkins this time, I should make a commotion and he's going to take off running. I think he forgot that his running ability is a bit compromised and we won't get very far!

We waited for about an hour to see Dr. Attar. He thought all looked really well but the drain had to stay for another week. Lee was really hoping to get that out, but I knew there was still so much fluid coming out (because I have to clean it two times a day!) that they would leave it in. As far as the infection, the cultures showed a staph infection. But it is hopefully a very low-grade infection that can be treated orally and not through a port. We will find out more when we see infectious disease docs. So for now . . . still no showers and one more week of the drain.

Last night he was really down in the dumps. He said he was tired of this whole ordeal and wanted his life back. He's been so amazing through this whole process. I reminded him what a strong patient he has been and he better not give up on me now. McNicey will not hear of it! Today I am heading up to Long Island to be with Tim. Lee is coming up tomorrow. He is stopping in NYC to take Cryder out to lunch for his birthday and then out to Long Island to see Tim. He hasn't seen Tim since before he got out of the hospital and is very eager to see him. I just know it will cheer him up to see both his boys.

This Father's Day, we all have a lot to celebrate! Including the return of Lee's hair. I referred to him as my chia pet. I told him the other day that his head looked like a kiwi fruit!! It's even showing some signs of darker hair too . . . not just gray!!

Hope you all have a great Father's Day weekend.

xoxox

When I picked Lee up at the train station, he was quite proud of himself for his journey to the city and then out to Long Island. He was full of stories about Cryder—which I was dying to hear, jealous that he got to see him and I didn't—but Lee was also very obviously excited to be on Long Island and finally seeing Tim again. My two warriors were reuniting.

We arrived at the house, and Lee quickly dropped his bags by the door and raced down the hall to see Tim. I loved seeing the two of them embrace and give each other a good pat on the back. Lee, of course, was still easily brought to tears, even at happy times. Tim, too, was visibly moved, seeing how much stronger his dad had become in the last few weeks.

Mom and Jack heard all the commotion in Tim's room and soon appeared in the doorway. Neither of them had seen Lee in a long time. Mom and Jack couldn't believe how well he looked. He'd regained some of his weight and looked great.

We caught up for a few minutes, and then we all disappeared to get dressed for dinner. I went back in to help Tim and was surprised to find he had managed to get himself dressed and ready. He looked so handsome in his ironed shorts (still couldn't wear pants over his leg), his button-down shirt, and his navy blue blazer. Lee came in to see if he could help, but now it was time for Tim to show off. He sat over the edge of the bed and, with his walker, maneuvered his way to the wheelchair. You could see that he was using every bit of strength he had, but he was determined to show us how far he had come. Lee watched with both a smile and a few tears.

An unfortunate pattern was developing in our lives. Just when everything seemed to be improving, something would go wrong. But these setbacks were not going to discourage us. Every positive step forward seemed to give me more hope. When a step backward occurred, it just made all of us more determined to fight back.

Monday morning, Tim had an appointment with Dr. Helfet where he was supposed to test putting weight on his left leg, and while I waited for Tim's call, I also waited for Lee's report from his infectious diseases doctor. Lee was still on antibiotics for his staph infection.

Tim's appointment with Dr. Helfet was first. I could still envision the first time Tim tried to lower his legs over the bed after the accident and could still hear his screams of pain. When he called to share the great news that all had gone well, a huge weight was lifted from my shoulders. The worry subsided momentarily. One down, one to go. Lee's news was not as positive. Still signs of infection, so the antibiotics would continue.

At the end of June, Lee and I celebrated thirty years together. What a milestone. We had the most wonderful evening, sitting on our back porch, reminiscing about the many amazing parts of our life, and the new phase ahead with the house we had just bought in Newport. It was magical when we fell in love, and after so many years together, I still felt like the luckiest woman alive.

I hope the same for my two sons. In fact, when Tim was still in the hospital in New York, we had one of our quiet moments together, just talking about life and how things change. Tim paused for a moment, then looked at me with those beautiful blue eyes that always captivate me and said, "Mom, I need to get a ring."

I wanted to jump out of my chair and hug him. "Oh yes, you do!" I said. "Gina is a remarkable woman, and you are so lucky to have found her. It's about time!" I was so excited, but we had to keep it a secret.

How, though, was Tim going to find a ring from a hospital bed in NYC? McNicey to the rescue again. I told Tim he should do some research online and then tell me the type of ring he'd like. We had a good friend with a wonderful jewelry store in Baltimore. On my next visit to the hospital, I arrived carrying a case filled with a dozen rings. I was a nervous wreck as the courier, sure that someone would jump me and grab the rings, but I delivered it safely to Tim, and he chose a stunning ring that he hid away until he was ready.

To propose, Tim insisted on taking Gina to her favorite place, Nantucket, which also happened to be where they'd met six years before. He was determined to get down on one knee to ask for her hand. What a hopeless romantic! I loved it. He was targeting the end of July for that to happen. It was so hard for me not to tell anyone, not even my mom, to whom I tell almost everything!

27

Summer Healing

Our first somewhat normal family event took place over the Fourth of July weekend on the North Shore of Long Island, where Lee and I had lived in our younger years. This year, John Smith had asked Lee to play with him in the golf tournament that weekend—a particularly good incentive for Lee to get strong enough to play three rounds of eighteen holes of golf in three days. Lee welcomed the challenge.

In the end, Lee didn't play his best golf, but he played and we all celebrated that. Tim usually participated in the softball tournament, which is more of a social event for his age group, with six teams and plenty of beer, but he obviously wouldn't be playing this time, so he insisted that Gina join in while he filled the role of team mascot. The club was nice enough to let Tim borrow a golf cart, which he drove very cautiously, so he could make his way out to the fields and watch from the sidelines. Everyone was thrilled to see him there.

Cryder played on a team, as well, and made sure he put on a good show for Tim. It was a spectacular weekend with lots of laughs and good times.

Subject: Could be the Last McNicey Report!
Our lives have changed so much since I last wrote.

On vacation in Rhode Island, Lee was rejuvenated, breathing in the sea air and so happy to be in his favorite place. His wound was still open and he was not able to dive into the ocean, but he insisted he was ready to start a routine of morning bike rides. The first day we biked together he could barely make it for ten minutes before turning around. By the end of the month he was able to ride for about forty-five minutes! We played golf every day for the first two weeks, and by the end of those two weeks Lee had graduated from riding in a cart to walking eighteen holes!!!! After many weeks of wound care, I finally gave him the green light to dive into that beautiful water. It just happened that Tim was up for the weekend and he too had been approved to go swimming, so they plunged into the ocean together. I don't know who had a bigger smile . . . Lee, Tim . . . or me!!!

And as for Tim: when he arrived in Newport, he climbed out of the car with ONE CRUTCH!! I couldn't believe it. He was walking on his foot!! The lump was still the same, it had not shrunk much and his foot was still very swollen, but he was walking! We had a great couple of days with him, but the most exciting news happened the following week.

On July 29, Tim took Gina to Nantucket, and although he did his best to get down on one knee (he couldn't quite make it) she still said YES!!! Yup, Tim and Gina are engaged!!! Tim had been planning this for over a month. (You can only imagine how difficult it was for me to keep a secret that long!!)

As I have said before, Tim had a lot of time to think over the past months and one thing was for certain, he was very lucky to have found someone as special as Gina, and there was no doubt he wanted to spend the rest of his life with her. She told me she was the happiest girl in the whole world, and so was I!!! Lee and I feel so lucky to have Gina join our family. Cryder is gaining a sister and couldn't be happier, plus Tim asked him to be his best man. Amazingly, within the last week, Tim's lump has suddenly begun to shrink and that has given us all a huge boost! He is hoping to be able to dance his famous moves by wedding time!

Just in case you all think I've forgotten about Cryder... he is doing great too. He finished his internship in New York and the two of us traveled up to Maine to visit Mom and Jack for a few days. We had many hours in the car and on the ferry and just hanging out together in our little cottage in Maine. I always cherish the time I have with my children. The one-on-ones, where you can just talk about nothing and everything.

Cryder shared so many thoughts about this past year, the good and the bad times. How helpless he felt being at school when he wanted to be in Baltimore with Lee or in New York with Tim. How amazing it has been to watch the two of them endure so much with incredible selfless-ness and determination. How worried he was about me being alone through it all. But I never was... I have had such incredible support from all of you and my amazing family.

Lee now has curls again, Tim is walking, Cryder is going back to UNC for one more semester and all is good... no, all is great, and Tim is getting married!!!

The DiPietros are back and we are now out from under our dark cloud!

Love to all of you, always.

What I didn't include in my email was that on our arrival in Rhode Island, I noticed that as much as Lee was gaining strength, I could not seem to shake the cobwebs. It was most apparent on my daily runs, when I couldn't seem to get any spring in my step. Each day, my legs felt like they were running in wet sand. I'd had runs like that many times over the years, but usually after a day or two and some extra rest

I could snap myself out of it. This time, though, it wasn't happening. All I wanted to do was go to the beach and sleep.

Despite my lack of energy, I still decided to run my usual half-marathon in West Virginia in mid-August. As I expected, I didn't have a great race, but that just made me determined to get back in gear, which finally became possible in September. Good thing too since Tim asked me to run the New York City Marathon, which I planned to do in November for both Tim and Lee, just as I had run a marathon for my sister Ames at the end of the past year. I couldn't believe all that had happened in that period of time.

I'd always hated the end of the summer. When I was young, it meant the end of the warm days we would enjoy in Newport, Rhode Island, and the start of school. When I was married and a mother, it meant the end of the special time our family spent with Mom and Jack in Vinalhaven, Maine—and the start of school for the boys. When the boys then went off to college, the end of August was even worse as I would watch them drive away with their cars loaded for their year away from home. I would hug them good-bye, choking back the tears. I was a big baby, as my boys would call me!

Lee, on the other hand, was thrilled to have me all to himself, and we loved meeting each other in the late afternoons for a quick nine holes of golf while the sun was going down. Lee loved to challenge my competitive spirit. Of course, I still had my running, and I was eager now to get back into training, although I felt as if I had, indeed, aged a bit in the last year.

28

Return to New York

Our lives were speeding up again. Lee was getting back to focusing on work and spending full days in the office. I was busy planning engagement parties and trying to get myself into marathon shape. Now that Tim and Lee were getting stronger by the day, I could afford to focus more attention on myself. I had a lot of work to do to get ready to run the New York Marathon.

Although I had reestablished the endurance part of racing, the speed part still seemed to be missing. The hardest part of training for me is the speed workout. It beats you up and breaks you down. And as you get older, it's harder to muster the strength to put yourself through a really rigorous workout of four to five miles of interval training—various combinations of a quarter mile or half mile at a 5k pace and a one mile at half-marathon pace. I dreaded these once-a-week workouts, but they had to be done, along with one day of tempo running where I run a half-marathon pace for forty-five minutes.

But I was most excited about the first of the engagement parties planned at Mom and Jack's house in Mill Neck at the end of September. On Saturday morning, before the party, we had a special moment planned. Tim and Lee had been in communication with the local fire department and the rescue team that had responded to Tim's accident. We planned to meet at the fire station, not only to talk with the lead guy on the team, but to give them a donation for saving Tim's life. When we were having breakfast that morning, I asked Tim if he thought he would remember what the guy looked like. We had never really talked about that before. He said he didn't think so, but he certainly remembered his name.

"What's that?" I asked.

"DiPietro!"

Crazy! I was stunned. He had never mentioned that before.

Lee, Tim, Gina, and I headed over to the fire station. As we climbed out of the car, a man in uniform appeared out of the open garage door. We were supposed to be meeting with the fire chief as well as John DiPietro. Lee stuck out his hand and asked, "Are you the chief?"

"No, I'm LieutenantJohn DiPietro."

We all sort of stopped in our tracks, not sure what to say for a second and then Tim said, "Hi, I'm Tim."

He said, "Yes, I remember you."

I started to shake his hand but stopped short. "I think I have to hug you . . . I don't know what to say. Thank you, thank you, we owe you so much." I was almost in tears again. It was such an overwhelmingly emotional moment for all of us to be able to finally thank the team who'd saved Tim.

Then a woman came from around the corner, pushing a stroller with an adorable little girl inside. Johnturned around and said, "Oh, this is my wife, Gina DiPietro."

"Wow . . . you are kidding!" Tim said. "This is my fiancée Gina, soon to be Gina DiPietro, too."

Now that was bizarre! We stood and chatted a while, reminiscing about the accident and listening to his rendition of the whole thing. One thing John wanted to know was who had put the tourniquet around Tim's leg?

Tim answered, "I did."

All John said was "Wow."

John added that when he got to the accident he only had a crew of rookies with him, and then he laughed and said the accident was a real eye-opener for them. John was the one who made the call for the helicopter, because the cops on the scene didn't think it was that bad. If he hadn't made that decision, things might have turned out very differently for Tim.

Listening to John tell the story about Tim's accident was also frightening. We learned how incredibly brave Tim had been and how amazing it was for him to have had the presence of mind to tourniquet his own leg and ultimately help save his own life.

The other amazing thing was John. I couldn't stop looking at him. He looked so much like Lee's deceased father, it was uncanny. John had the same round face and shaved head and was about the same height and build with a wonderfully warm smile. Both the name and the resemblance were truly eerie.

After we delivered the check and when I was alone in the car with Lee, I said, "I have to tell you, I couldn't believe how much John DiPietro looked like your father."

Tears immediately welled up in his eyes. He was quiet for a minute and then said, "He came back to save Tim."

With all my heart I believe that is true. Forever we will be grateful, and I will never forget the man who looked so much like Lee's father.

The September night of Tim and Gina's engagement party was a huge celebration. It felt like a return to Mom and Jack's old Christmas parties with the front hall and living room filled with guests bearing gifts and huge smiles. Gina looked absolutely radiant, and of course Tim looked so handsome. It seemed everyone wanted to be a part of such a welcome celebration. Tim and Gina were on cloud nine, and it was great to see.

The period leading up to the NYC Marathon was incredibly hectic. In between traveling from Baltimore to New York to see Tim, from Baltimore to New Jersey for an engagement party, and from Baltimore to Philadelphia for the Philadelphia Half-Marathon, I was in full training mode in preparation for the marathon. I was very pleased with the

Philadelphia race, where I finished with a time of 1:25:48, eight minutes faster than the West Virginia race, and it showed that my hard
work had paid off.

Just a week before the marathon, however, we were waiting for
scan results on Lee from Dr. Attar. By Friday, on the eve of the marathon, we'd still heard nothing. I wish I could blame the results of the
race on my anxiety, but I don't think that was entirely the case. I think
more than anything I was still pretty rundown from the last several
months of our lives, and I'd had difficulty doing the speed training.

I had added pressure too, racing as an invited sub-elite runner,
which is an honor, especially in a big league race like the New York
Marathon. Plus, I'd dedicated it to Lee and Tim, so I didn't want to
let them down. Let's just say that I wasn't going into the race with the
level of confidence I wanted.

Nonetheless, I was happy to be back in New York City doing what
I love. The city was in full swing. Energy was everywhere. Cryder and
Tim would be at the marathon, along with Lee and other members of
my family. I was so excited to have all of them there to cheer me on.

It was a cold windy day, not my favorite kind of running. I started
out just as planned, running a 6:30-minute mile pace. I was amazed at
how comfortable and smooth I felt despite the strong headwinds. I was
hoping to run the first half in under one hour and thirty minutes. At the
half-marathon mark I was well under my desired time, coming through
at 1:27:30. I still felt strong, but the cold wind was beginning to wear
me down, making my bare quads feel stiff.

As I ran over the Queensboro 59th Street Bridge at mile fifteen, I
began to feel that dreaded fatigue settle in, far too early in the race. My
pace began to slow and I began my usual conversations with myself.
Come on, keep your legs moving, stay light on your feet, drink, try using some
power gels. Anything to get to the finish. *Focus on the runners ahead, stay*
with them.

I struggled and even resorted to walking a few times at the water
stations during the last four miles, but I was driven by the crowds and
encouraged to continue. With about two miles to go, I could hear my

family's voices rising above the other wildly cheering spectators in Central Park. Somehow they had managed to get to another spot along the course, and hearing their voices gave me a jolt and reminded me why I was here.

Come on Lee, reach deep, find the strength to finish strong. The spectators were lifting my spirits, and it was thrilling to hear so many people shouting and cheering—even more thrilling when it was over! I had made it. It may not have been pretty, but I had made it. I was disappointed with my 3:08 finishing time, but I later heard that racing times were slower for many of the runners due to the conditions.

Lee asked me if I was upset about my finish. Yes, I was disappointed, but when reviewing events of the last year, I was really happy to just be there, running again, and having both Lee and Tim alive and feeling healthy. They had, by the way, walked clear across town from 1st Avenue to the finish in Central Park, where I could hear their shouting above the other voices. Now, if we could just get positive test results for Lee, that would make me more ecstatic than any race possibly could. However, a note from my mother to our friends and family made me exceedingly happy and helped assuage my disappointment over the race:

> Brewster, his kids, and I were at the NYC Marathon with the DiPietro contingent, and I cannot describe the thrill of seeing Lee racing up 1st Avenue towards us all, waving as she swept past us with those long graceful and DETERMINED strides! I have to admit to the sting of a few tears in my eyes and a burst of pride in my heart. She ran a 3:08, which I think is pretty good after the tribulations of the past year.
> xoxoxo
> Mother Nina

It wasn't until Tuesday morning during our appointment with Dr. Attar that we heard the scan results. To be exact, he said, "You are cancer free!" Words we were dying to hear, and of course that was the greatest gift he could have given us. Now it was our turn to present him with a thank you gift.

You might think it an odd choice, but we'd done some research and discovered that quite a lot of surgeons are "gamers." Apparently, it improves their dexterity, obviously a much needed skill for surgery. Dr. Attar was an enthusiastic "Xbox-er." When Lee handed him the new Xbox, he was visibly stunned. "No one's ever done that before," he said, which added to how wonderful we felt at that moment.

Once Dr. Attar left, I flew into Lee's arms and we hugged and cried. Emotions at such times can be so raw and powerful. I felt very lucky to have such a courageous man.

Though scans would be repeated every three months for two years, Dr. Attar had said he felt pretty confident Lee would be healthy and strong for a long time to come. And after one more surgery for Tim on the first of December, I hoped we could steer clear of hospitals for a long while.

After the marathon, Lee and I were anxious to get back to the warmth of Delray and have the boys join us for Thanksgiving. I couldn't believe how much had happened in the last year. Of course I thought of Ames, having lost her a year ago at this time, but wanted to stay focused on the positives. All of our friends in Florida were amazed that Lee looked like his old self, with hair thicker and curlier than ever, and they applauded how well Tim seemed to be doing, as if nothing had ever happened to either of them. We truly had much to be thankful for.

Thursday we all went to the beach, a gorgeous, warm day. Tim was a little self-conscious about his leg, but the turquoise blue ocean was luring the boys in. There were rough but perfect waves for body surfing. When Tim was a child, he spent all day in the water, catching waves and just getting rolled in the surf. Now he appeared hesitant to go in.

Cryder, being very protective of his brother, quietly followed alongside Tim, not to make him feel like an invalid, but ready to grab him if he needed help. It really warmed my heart to watch this unfold. As they entered the waves, Tim reached out and put his hand on Cryder's shoulder to steady himself. Of course, I was watching Tim like a hawk, aware that being unable to point your toes (as Tim couldn't) is a lot like dragging an anchor when you're swimming. So when the first wave came and Tim tried to catch it, his head looked like a lobster buoy being swept over by a wave. (Sorry Tim, not that your head really looks like a lobster buoy!) I saw his expression change with the realization that he wouldn't be able to catch a wave the way he used to. Cryder saw it too, and the next thing I knew they were wading in the water, talking, then they both flipped onto their backs and called out that they were practicing swim therapy as they laughed and kicked together. Thank you, Cryder!

But the next day, Tim, being one who never gives up, gave another attempt at body surfing. Again, Cryder helped him in. The waves were a bit rougher this time, so Lee took Tim's other side. Wish I had gotten a photo of that. Really choked me up to see the two of them surrounding Tim. First Tim floated for a while, assessing the situation, while Cryder threw himself into the waves, doing his best to entertain his brother. There is nothing Cryder likes more than to make Tim laugh!

I saw Tim eyeing the surf and the next thing I knew he had launched himself again, with arms moving quickly and powerfully. He managed to catch a short ride before being engulfed in the wave, but it was definitely a victory!

29

Beating the Odds

Christmas 2010 was the end of a nightmarish year, and I was preparing for the best Christmas ever. I wanted to spoil my men with everything I had! We decided to resume our old tradition of jumping in the car Christmas morning—of course, after we had opened our stockings and gifts to each other—and heading north to Mom and Jack's to celebrate a very special year with them and the rest of my family. Mom was particularly happy we were "coming home" because she and Jack had been so intertwined in our year of disasters, and they wanted to ring in a new era with us.

Mom had set the dining room table beautifully. I felt like a wide-eyed child gazing at a room filled with gifts and sparkling candlelight. It was a special Christmas; that was for sure. When Mom stood to make her usual Christmas dinner toast, the room grew silent. She praised both Lee and Tim for their strength and bravery, not forgetting to congratulate Cryder for graduating, and saying that she never believed it would happen! Of course, she was teasing him. She finished her toast, saying how proud she was of me, too, for keeping my head high and taking care of my family.

I never give toasts, but something propelled me to stand up. I had to thank my family and particularly Mom, Jack, and Brewster for taking Tim in and caring for him. We never would have gotten through the whole ordeal without them. I was in my usual seat, right next to

Jack—the seat of honor. I stood up from my chair to make my special toast, and when I turned to face Jack and thank him, I saw the tears brimming in his eyes. Here is this man of steel, a strong man in every sense of the word. I have never seen him shed a tear, and there it was about to spill over. That did me in, and through my sobs and shaky voice I proclaimed I was obviously not as strong as everyone thought I was, but I had to thank all of them from the bottom of my heart.

Sometime during this whole scene, Tim had risen from his seat and stood next to me, his arms around me, holding me up. Then the two of us hugged Jack. It was a release of so many worries, a cleansing of all the fears.

Jack simply said, with his shaky voice, "That is what family does."

I had hoped that Christmas would be nothing but a joyful weekend, but in the midst of everything we discovered that Tim's leg was very infected. I had nightmares of the infection working its way into the bone, because of something that had happened to my sister Nini when she was a teenager. She got an infection that traveled through her blood stream and settled in her shinbone. The infection had festered for a while, but no one knew it and she nearly lost her leg. The doctors had only a matter of hours to save it. This memory haunted me. We had all worked so hard to save Tim's leg, and I could tell that Tim was worried, too, but luckily he got an appointment with his doctor in New York City on Monday.

Mother Nature was up to her old tricks again, though, and New York was covered with snow that morning. Nevertheless we were determined to deliver Tim into the city for his appointment, and somehow we made it. As we thought, an infection was present, and the screws in the ankle were suspected as the source. Removing the screws would hopefully clear this up but they felt it could wait until the surgery, which wasn't scheduled until February 23.

Another surprise came as a result of Tim's appointment with Dr. Helfet. Tim had X-rays taken and they showed that the left tibia, where they'd removed the plate and twenty some odd screws, was "settling." Whatever that meant! If you looked at his X-rays (which Tim immediately emailed) you could see the middle of the tibia almost making a V, pushing towards the front of his shin. Dr. Helfet felt it was important to go in as soon as possible and re-rod the tibia before it pushed out any farther. They moved his surgery up to January 26. I was grateful for that as I hated the thought of waiting until late February to deal with the infection. Of course I would fly to New York to be there again for yet another surgery. I had to be there, in person, to watch over Tim.

Despite the forecasted snow for New York and expected delays, I arrived at Hospital for Special Surgery, to the familiar waiting room. During the surgery, when Dr. Helfet found me to give his report, I hadn't even started to pace yet. Everything sounded good. I know it seems silly, but one of the biggest questions for Tim was: would he ski again? There was so much more to worry about, like: Will he walk okay? Will the infection ever go away? Are there more complications that should concern us? But the skiing thing was something that meant a great deal to Tim; it meant he could have something of a normal life. And it was his passion, which I could definitely relate to. If you took my running away from me, what would I become?

I wish Gina and I could have gone together to deliver the good news to Tim, but I had to do it on my own while Gina was stuck at work. Standing at his bedside, I could see his eyes searching mine as I relayed Dr. Helfet's report. I couldn't contain the smile that crept across my face as I told him the news he was desperate to hear but was afraid to ask.

"Yes, you will ski again!" I said, wanting to hug him forever and tell him how brave he was and how proud I was of him. It was clearly a victory for him. He'd beaten the odds. A doctor had once told him he would probably never walk again without a brace, but now he could even dream of skiing. The tears escaped down his cheeks once again while his smile stretched across his face, matching mine.

I had not been prepared to deal with the amount of snow in New York, but I couldn't resist a run in Central Park. There was hardly anyone there; the branches were filled with snow and a fresh white blanket lay on the ground. It was worth every step climbing over the snow banks as I made my way into the park. The other "crazy runners" in Central Park were beaming, just like me.

Epilogue

Throughout the rest of winter of 2011, I watched Lee grow stronger, and although Tim suffered a few more setbacks with infections and possible surgeries, we navigated our way through the ups and downs. Sadly on the day after Valentine's Day, we received a phone call that Lee's mother had suffered a stroke but died peacefully in her sleep. Lee was devastated. He'd lost his father years earlier; now his mother was gone too, and so close on the heels of his own recovery.

In April, another bit of devastating news rocked us when the father of Cryder's best friend at UNC died of cancer. He'd been diagnosed the year before Lee, and we'd all watched Michael battle this horrible disease with so much courage. A great deal of admiration and camaraderie had formed between the two dads, as they simultaneously fought their cancer on Senior Day, the two of them sat together in the shade. Friends in good times and bad.

For several days after Michael died, Lee fell into depression. He was so sad and felt horribly guilty that he'd made it and Michael hadn't. At the funeral, Michael's son spoke about the wonderful memories he had of his father and what an incredible man he was. All the while, Lee wept silently, and I'm sure he was thinking that could have been him. Cryder was seated on Lee's other side and I imagine he was thinking the same. It reminded us again how precious life can be and how quickly things can change.

Spring was approaching, and I could see signs of my garden coming to life. I so enjoy digging my hands into the earth and preparing the soil for all the flowers. The buds on the trees were gaining size, and I was anticipating the beautiful burst of cherry blossoms. I couldn't wait for the next signs of life to explode. Wedding plans were coming together, which meant it was time to take a trip to Nantucket to see the choices being made. Something uplifting and happy to replace the sadness of winter.

Subject: Lee and Tim 1 year later

Oh, yes . . . it is your lucky day!! McNicey is back and this time it will be a wrap. The last report! I have been trying to figure out when to end these reports, and although Lee and Tim will still be dealing with doctors and tests, I figure now is the time to end. May 2 marked the one year anniversary when Lee's life was about to begin again and Tim's life hung in the balance. Lee's tumor was removed on May 3 and the cancer was gone . . . for Tim, the battle had just begun.

As May 2 approached this year, I was in a funny state of mind. So much has happened that we are all so grateful for, but a year ago this same weekend began a nightmare I will never forget. Again, like last year, Gina was in DC at her annual event and Tim was with the boys. This year, though, Tim is a very different man. He was doing a lot of reminiscing and thinking too. As difficult as it has been, and the fact that his leg will always be a challenge, he knows how lucky he is to have his leg and his life.

We laughed about me being such a worrying mom, but he understands that some things will never change! In fact, I was counting my lucky stars because they returned safely from his bachelor party. Cryder and the other groomsmen decided to kidnap Tim and take him to Puerto Rico for the weekend. Couldn't they have just gone to Florida? I threatened several of them with their lives and told them if anything happened, they would have to answer to me . . . McMeany!! Actually, Cryder was pretty funny about having to take care of the lot of them!! He said it was quite the babysitting job!! At least that's his side of the story! The rest I don't want to know!!

The following Friday, we were meeting with Tim, Gina, and her parents in Nantucket to explore all the wedding venues and go over plans. We visited the church and I pictured Tim and Gina saying their vows this coming October. It was a gorgeous weekend in Nantucket and Gina had everything all planned, including a sunset ride out to the Great Point where they got engaged.

We brought a bottle of wine (well, maybe a couple of bottles!) and celebrated their coming wedding. It was so warming to see how happy the two of them are.

We decided we should try to take a group picture, but of course no one else was out there. It's a very remote spot at that time of night. So Tim set his camera (with the self-timer) on the roof of the car, while we all stood posing and ready. Not thinking . . . we had Tim set up the camera, and as it started to beep and count down, Tim tried to scurry from the car to stand with all of us. He was moving amazingly quickly and we all started laughing as Tim ran and said, "Who picked the handicapped guy to run into the picture?!" But he made it and I was thrilled to see he could almost run with a hop and get there. Hmmm . . . maybe a run for charity for him . . . just kidding!

The following week, Tim came back to Baltimore for a few nights. One exciting thing that has happened in Tim's life (well, we hope it will be exciting!) is that he left his job in NYC and is now working with Lee. He'll still be working and living in the city, just opening up a satellite office up there. So he had to come down to Baltimore for a few days of training. The first night home, we were sitting in the kitchen and Tim picked his foot up and rested it on the coffee table. He had taken his compression sock off to show us his leg. The first thing I noticed was the size of his foot and ankle. For the first time in a year, I could actually see the bones in his toes. I was suddenly hopeful that someday he would actually have a close to normal looking foot again. The flap had also gone down since the last time we saw it. Incredible progress.

Now for Lee. A week ago Tuesday, Lee had his one-year CT scan and MRI. I was in New York and had requested that Dr. Attar send me an email. When I opened it the only words I remember were: "Good news, the scans were all clean." I guess I'll always worry a little before I hear that phrase. Tears literally popped out of my eyes while Tim and Gina were watching me wondering what the heck was going on.

"Dad's scans," I said, "they're all clean!" We all high-fived and I composed myself as I quickly forwarded the email to Lee. For now, the beast has been slaughtered and Lee is as healthy as ever. Maybe a little too healthy!! Ha Ha!! But McNicey is working on that, too, if you know what I mean!! Back to boot camp for my man!

So as I said at the beginning of this email, this will be my last report, I hope!! I can't thank you all enough for all the emails, the cards, the incredible support you have given us all over the past year. It has certainly been a roller-coaster ride for us and it's time to get off!! I am hoping to finish my book next week . . . a good place for this to end . . . one year later. So if you ever miss hearing from McNicey, and, if I'm lucky . . . maybe a book will land on the shelf! All our best to all of you . . . have a wonderful summer and much love from all of us.

xoxox

A Special Tribute

Sometimes there is someone who comes into your life and changes you forever. My stepfather was one of those people. He was a man's man, a former Marine, as mysterious and smooth as James Bond and as clever and resourceful as MacGyver. He and my mother had a true love story. They fell in love when each had already committed to another life. Although they tried to resist the attraction, their love was too strong. Jack married my mother and took in her five daughters, raising us as his own.

I adored this man and followed him everywhere I could. I was the tomboy who loved to have him teach me how to throw a baseball or shoot skeet. He had a reputation as an excellent marksman and, when skeet-shooting, could handle a gun with a one smooth swing of the barrel.

The stories he told about his life were never ending and left me with my mouth open, in awe of the adventures he had. He traveled to Africa several times, starting his own safari outfit. I was never lucky enough to go to Africa with him, but I relived all his adventures through the amazing photographs he took. He could tell a story like no other person, as you plunged into the picture he painted, living it over and over again through his eyes. Recapping his days in Korea, where he served as a Marine, he told tales of bravery, camaraderie, and loyalty. He was quick to dismiss his heroics, though, never asking for any praise. Respect? There was no one I respected more.

A year after Lee and I were married, we moved back to Long Island from Boston and built a house on property we bought from Jack. Despite our invasion of his woods and his privacy, Jack knew how happy our move would make Mom and so agreed to let us settle in next door.

When Tim was born, Jack welcomed him as his own grandchild. He was one of the first to visit me in the hospital when he was born. Although he pretended to not like babies and made it very clear that no crying babies were encouraged to visit, I caught him several times eyeing our tiny child with a secret smile. As Tim grew and then Cryder arrived, the boys were also intrigued by this giant of a man. But they knew there were boundaries and strict rules. We threatened them with the wrath of "umps," as they called him, if they misbehaved. They both were a little afraid of him, but Tim was quick to realize that Jack had a soft heart and he wiggled his way into it.

Jack quietly took my boys under his wing, teaching them how to sail a boat and respect the sea, handle a gun and not use it as a toy, behave like gentlemen and always look someone in the eye when you shook their hand, respect all people, no matter who they were, live life with open eyes, and take your licks when you deserved it, always appreciating the lesson you learned. Of course, I had learned these lessons from him, too, but seeing my boys absorb all they could from Jack's presence was a precious gift.

I am still processing why things happened the way they did this last year and a half. I don't know if I will ever make sense of it, but somehow I gained strength when I needed to, and I truly feel I learned how to be brave in the face of danger from Jack. "Be strong," I would tell myself, "be a Marine."

When Lee was first diagnosed with cancer, my head was spinning. I knew I would find comfort and strength calling home. Jack was always calm in the face of disaster; he could always make things better. When I spoke to him on the phone, just hearing his voice and having him tell me we had great doctors and it would be OK convinced me it would be so. He assured me he would be there when I needed him. "Call anytime, Kiddo. Let us know if there is anything we can do."

The first number I dialed when Tim had his accident was Jack's. He was in his car in route to the hospital without a seconds delay, beating the helicopter to the hospital. There he stood guard, watching over Tim and waiting to consult with the doctors. I had faith that if anyone could fix this mess, it would be Jack. After that first horrible night, I later found out that Jack wasn't so sure this time he could fix it. When Mom flew to Baltimore to bring me back to Tim, Jack stood watch in the ICU at the Nassau University Medical Center. There was nowhere for him to sit, so he stood at the foot of Tim's bed, watching over him as the machines beeped and nurses hovered while Tim slept unconsciously. Jack was there; he would protect Tim and send him his strength. When I flew back to Long Island and met up with Jack on route to the hospital, it became apparent that Tim was far worse than I imagined. Jack looked deep into my eyes and my soul, willing me to be strong and fight by Tim's side.

Jack never went back to the hospital after those first two days in the ICU, next seeing Tim only when we brought him home to Jack's house a month later. I think Jack feared the worst, and maybe kept himself clear knowing he had already given Tim everything he had. But when we arrived at the house in Long Island and maneuvered Tim out of the car, Jack was there, waiting, his hands outstretched to help Tim. There, he took charge, holding onto Tim's wheelchair, guiding him back into his care, not wanting to let go.

For the next month, Jack nursed Tim back, caring for his wounds, helping him gain strength, encouraging him both physically and mentally. The days and nights Tim spent with Jack would be cherished memories. Tim became privy to all of Jack's life stories and his life lessons. Jack took my son in, cared for him, loved him, and taught him how to be brave in the face of danger.

Sadly, as I wrote the last "McNicey" report in May, a year after Lee's surgery and Tim's accident, Jack was in trouble then, and this was going to be hard to fix. I purposely didn't mention anything about Jack's illness in that report as we wanted to keep it private until we knew what we were dealing with.

In April, Jack started experiencing excruciating pain in his back and reluctantly saw his doctor. He was diagnosed with a fractured vertebra, given strong pain medication, and told to stay quiet and let it heal. For three weeks, he suffered with this pain, hardly able to walk and too uncomfortable to sit. Eventually he was taking such high doses of pain medication that we all became concerned. I remember telling him that the dose he was taking was way too much and that he should go back and have this checked further. He claimed he just had a high tolerance for pain medication.

Then Mom called me one morning in an absolute panic. As we moms tend to do, she had this horrible nightmare. She dreamt that something was terribly wrong with Jack. She was terrified the pain in his back was being caused by a tumor growing. Lee's diagnosis had made cancer so real to Mom that it had become an underlying fear. You never know when cancer can strike. She was becoming increasingly frustrated with the doctor who had only done an X-ray on Jack's back and no other tests. I told her, from what we had learned, that he should have an MRI. Jack, of course, refused saying his doctor was handling it and she should stay out of it. I told Mom to call the doctor, explain her fears and insist the doctor order an MRI. That way the suggestion was coming from the doctor, not her.

"Listen," I said, "you have to rule things out. He needs this test. Don't worry."

Easier said than done. I, too, had terrible fears that this was something worse. Jack was now in such great pain that he could barely walk down the hallway from his bedroom to the kitchen. The only place he found some degree of comfort was on his back in bed

Mom had learned to be persistent, though, from witnessing all that Lee and I had dealt with in the hospitals. She called Jack's doctor and was victorious: an MRI was scheduled for Thursday. Good for her!

On Friday morning, I was waiting anxiously to hear from Mom on the day the MRI results were due. Lee and I were in Florida on a business trip. So while Lee was in meetings, I went on my usual morning run and then headed to the fitness center to ride the bike because I couldn't sit still.

When the call came, I rushed out of the fitness center with my phone pressed hard to my ear. It only took me a second to realize our fears were right; the sound of Mom's voice said it all. I knew before her words ended: it was cancer. There was a mass on Jack's lung that had grown into his spine, fracturing the spine and putting pressure on the nerve.

My breath escaped me and I sank onto the brick wall. *Oh, God, not again.* The tables had turned. Just a few months before, Mom had been the first person I had called when we learned that Lee's lump was a sarcoma. It was my turn now to be her shoulder to cry on. This couldn't be happening. And here I was in Florida, so far away.

In two days, though, we would be flying to Newport on our way to meet Tim, Gina, and Gina's parents for a weekend in Nantucket to finalize plans for the wedding and see where they would be married. I told Mom that as soon as I got to Newport I would jump in the car and drive to Long Island, be there to hold her hand and help her with where they went from here. I knew how overwhelming this news was and how hard it was to digest and take the next steps forward. "No," she said. The weekend was important to Tim and Gina, and there was nothing I could do that she couldn't handle herself. Mom is amazingly strong, and I knew she would take charge, but I also knew she needed a shoulder to lean on. Luckily, Brewster was there, helping to take care of Jack and keeping their spirits up as only Brewster could do. But, of course, Brewster was in a tailspin too. This was his dad, and he was suffering.

Mom called me daily, reporting all the information the doctors were giving her. I was her source of knowledge; I'd been through this before. And I was beginning to fear the worst. I knew from Lee's initial meetings with his doctors that the biggest danger with a sarcoma would be if the cells broke away. They had explained that the first place the cells tend to travel was the lungs, and, if that happened, it would not be good. So I was more than aware of what it meant when the cancer was in the lungs.

The other thing that scared me was Jack had this persistent cough for the last couple of years. It took him months of dealing with this cough before he eventually gave in and had a lung scan. Jack had smoked a pipe for years, and the fear of lung cancer was a given. The scan showed he had a spot on his lung that "had to be watched." As was typical of him, Jack shrugged it off, saying he was just getting old and these things happened.

The cough persisted, but never really got worse; it was just always there. I knew he had been particularly worried about this cough the previous summer. He made a strange comment to me at a dinner just before he left for Maine for the summer, jokingly saying he wouldn't be around much longer. He said that often, making light of the aging process, perhaps trying to prepare himself for the inevitable. But this time his comment struck me differently. I wondered if he was trying to tell me something. Mom had become so accustomed to the cough and assumed he was in tune with his health and continuing with his scans.

Lee and I had a few days in Newport before heading to Nantucket. My morning runs were my chance to beg God once again, this time to save Jack. I spent hours trying to make sense of another blow to our family.

"Why us again? Please, I know we've asked for so many favors, but please, God, help us get through this again. Please give Mom the strength she needs. Please don't take Jack from us." I apologized for asking for another favor after all He had helped us get through.

I had been in Newport for four days and was in constant contact with Mom. Things were spiraling out of control. They had done a surgery on Jack a few weeks ago to try to relieve the pressure on his nerve in his spine, but it wasn't working. He was in terrible pain. They had already set up his chemo and radiation treatments that were to begin immediately. Mom was distraught. She couldn't stand watching him in such pain. The doctors ordered a PET scan to see where the cancer had traveled and would review the results with Mom, Jack, and Brewster on Friday morning.

That morning, I ran and then paced and paced, dug in the garden, and waited for her call. Finally the ring, and the caller ID said *Mom*. When I answered the phone, there was a muffled, barely audible

"Lee" and then the crying. I felt that familiar feeling of the blood rushing from my head, and my limbs going weak. *Oh, please, no.* But this time the cancer had traveled too far. It had metastasized into the bone. I knew what this meant, and so did she. Brewster was there with her but all I wanted to do was hold her in my arms and let her cry. But Mom being Mom, she pulled herself together, saying over and over, "I'm OK, I'm OK."

"I'm coming home," I said, but she was adamant that I go with Tim and Gina to Nantucket. There was nothing I could do. It was a moment I will never forget. It was like a dream, but so real and one I had floated through before.

When I picked up Lee at the airport in Providence a few hours later, I was still numb. It took me some time to find the words to tell him the news. I knew how hard he would take this: cancer rearing its head again, this time to a man who acted as his father in so many ways. Lee was devastated.

We put on our best smiles over the weekend in Nantucket deciding not to tell Tim and Gina and ruin their special weekend. I'm not sure if it was the right decision. Later when I told the boys and Gina, they were distraught. They had seen Jack a few weeks earlier and knew he was in a lot of pain, but they never imagined it would come to this. We had been through enough this year. This was unimaginable.

The cancer had taken hold and traveled relentlessly through his body. I can't tell you how brave Jack was as he faced this horrible disease. Mom and Brewster were by his side every step with their brave faces. I was not far behind whenever they needed me. As soon as I got home from Nantucket, I was on my way to Long Island, that familiar route in my white chariot.

Jack was a skeleton of his former self. He had not eaten any solid food since the lung cancer was found. Mom was frustrated that he refused to eat, and she tried all his favorite recipes, but I understood: He was taking control of what he could control. He was going to live life on his own terms and not let cancer dictate how he lived. It was heartbreaking. He was going downhill fast. Mom's control was spiraling away too, but she was hanging on with everything she had.

The cancer stormed through his body in a matter of weeks, and the fight was over. It happened so fast. How could you even have time to think about what was happening? No time for denial, it just took over and sped away with another precious life. I'm quite sure that his choice to refuse solid food accelerated the process by weakening his strength to fight. It was his way of saving all of us from watching him suffer. An amazingly selfless man to the end, his family's pain was so much more important than his own. His death came on Memorial Day. How fitting was that?

A month and a half after Jack's death, I accompanied Mom to Maine. Mom and Jack had spent every summer on their island in Maine for the last forty-five years. It was their special place, somewhere they could go back in time and forget about troubles and live a simple life. After much thought, Mom decided she would continue her summer tradition without Jack by her side. But it was going to be tough to travel by ferry to their cherished home and enter their house without him. I volunteered to be there and hold her hand.

As we approached the island and the ferry neared its landing, Mom's eyes filled with tears and her lip began to quiver. Here was a woman, strong-willed and determined, one I admired beyond words—how could I help her heal, help her get through this ache in her heart? I hugged her tight and told her it would be OK. Jack was there, at the house, waiting to welcome us, I just knew it.

We arrived at the house and climbed the long back stairs, carrying armloads of bags. I felt an ache in my heart as I opened the back door. And there on the porch, overlooking the thoroughfare, was Jack's favorite chair. It would stay empty now. We both glanced at it knowing it would be so. We unpacked, settled in, and met on the porch for an evening glass of wine in Jack's honor. As we sat and talked about all that had happened and how Jack would be there watching over Mom in everything she did, an amazing double rainbow appeared on the horizon. We both watched as it grew from the sea to the sky, and we found comfort in it as a sign from Jack: he was there; everything was going to be OK.

Later that evening, in the quiet of the night under millions of stars filling the sky, I told Mom how guilty I felt about all the favors God had given us for Lee and Tim. I had used them all up for us and there had been none left for Jack. I confided in her that I had a suspicion Jack knew his cancer was there long before it was diagnosed but didn't want anyone to know. He would silently suffer, knowing it would take him in the long run. Mom said she thought the same thing and had been afraid to talk about it.

Then she told me a story. She told me about the day Lee was in Hopkins, in surgery, the day after Tim's accident. She told me how Jack had gone to be with Tim in the ICU. There he stood at the foot of Tim's bed, watching over him, willing him to live. He had called Mom and told her that Tim was in really bad shape and that he was so worried. He said we needed to get back to Tim as quickly as possible. Mom said she believed that Jack made a deal with God that day, that he told God to take him instead of Tim. If someone had to go, take him. Jack was not a religious man by any means, so I am not sure how he might have conversed with God, but I, too, believe he saved my son that day.

I will never be able to tell Jack how much I love him, how grateful I am for all he was to me and my husband and my children. What an amazing man he was—brave, heroic, humble, generous, honest, trustworthy, and loving in a very quiet way. He was more than a father to me, and he was an incredible grandfather to our sons. For all he was and all he will be to us forever, I pay tribute to him here.

As for Mom, the healing process will be long and hard. But, like me, she is a runner and has been since she ran her first race in Baltimore with me in 1994. And now at the age of seventy-eight, she still runs her three miles several times a week. I know those runs will be her time to think, to search for answers and to heal. With each run, she will feel the pounding of her heart and her lungs burning, reminding her she is alive and strong as we all go forward in life.

A Special Thank You

Cancer is a frightful word. As is suicide. And a life-threatening accident with a long recovery can be hard for people to deal with. What meant so very much to me and to my husband and sons were those family and friends who were not frightened or intimidated by any of this, but instead chose to stand with us as we confronted it all. They did not let us walk this tightrope alone but delivered food, lent an ear, wrote uplifting notes, sent encouraging cards, and were always offering to help. To all our friends and family who helped us in our darkest moments, from my sister's death to our crises with Lee and Tim, we are forever thankful.

During Lee's fight with cancer, I struggled to keep my thoughts positive and a smile on my face. I never wanted him to see the fear in my eyes, only the fight. I received so much support in that effort from the many who directly helped Lee in his battle—his doctors, nurses, therapists, and aides. I will never be able to thank Dr. Attar and Dr. Frassica enough for giving Lee his life back. Their dedication and that of their staff to helping other people is beyond admirable. We are so grateful for their skill, faith, and compassion.

When your own child is badly injured, the pain cuts even deeper. Tim's accident coming on the cusp of Lee's recovery was a severe blow to us all. His injuries were grave. Would he walk? Would he live? With Lee in the hospital and Cryder at school, all I could do was go forward—not give up and make sure Tim didn't give up. But I had help from so many. I could not have survived that first week with Tim in the ICU if it hadn't been for Gina and my family and all of Tim's friends and my friends who rallied around us. Gina was faced with losing the man she loved, and never have I seen someone so caring, nurturing, gentle, and kind dealing with so much more than she ever bargained for. To all of Tim's friends who encircled his bed, urging him to stay strong and heal, and to our friends who gathered in the halls of the ICU lending what they could to help us keep Tim from fading away, I owe you so much. To Mom and Edie who held my hand in the ICU, keeping me standing strong while you struggled yourselves, I thank you from the bottom of my heart.

I will also be forever grateful to Lt. DiPietro and his EMT team for their quick response to the accident, to the amazing ER doctors who saved Tim's leg, and to the ICU team that nursed Tim through some very rough days. I will never be able to say thank you enough to Dr. Helfet and Dr. Gael and their incredible team of doctors, nurses, and staff. The kindness, compassion, encouragement, and support from every single one of Tim's doctors, nurses, and PT's was unending. But they gave Tim more than great medical care—they gave him hope.

Without the love and support of so many family members, our battles could never have been won. Their outpouring of love through so many emails, letters, and phone calls lifted our spirits. The heartfelt encouragement and support of my other sisters, Edie, Kitty, Nini, Wendy, and Leigh, meant the world to me. And Mom, Jack, and Brewster have my undying gratitude for their unending love and support in nursing Tim and helping him walk again. Brewster filled in for Gina when she could not be with Tim and spent every morning helping Tim shower and dress, pushing him to get his strength back. Jack stood by Tim and gave him his courage. Mom was my rock in so many ways, guiding me through the heartache even as she ached for all. I got my strength from her.

Mostly, I must thank my three men. Without them, I am nothing. They give me a reason to live. Cryder suffered along with his father as he saw the cancer tearing him down, then stood bravely as he almost lost his brother. He felt helpless so far away, but never did he let us know his fears and, whenever he could, he made sure he was there to wrap his big arms around me and let me know he wouldn't let me fall. Perhaps more than anything, he kept me smiling through some very rough moments, as did Tim. Their sense of humor kept me alive. Tim's frequent phone calls and emails during Lee's chemo and radiation confirmed that he was with us in spirit even if he was hundreds of miles away.

Tim and Lee must be thanked above all, though, for their incredible bravery and their will to fight, for their trust and their love. Both of them amazed everyone with their patience, courage, strong wills, and uncomplaining spirit. People tell me, "You got your men through this. If it hadn't been for you, things would have been different." But they are wrong. Lee and Tim fought harder than anyone will ever know. I was only their coach and cheerleader. It was their fight and their victory, and we are a family united in celebration of that victory.

Acknowledgments

I would like to first thank those who read my "McNicey Reports" that encouraged me to write this book, suggesting it might help others face hurdles in their life. Without their insistence, this book would not have been written.

Thank you to my agent Frederica Friedman who pushed me to make this a better story and who introduced me to Skyhorse Publishing.

To Julia Abramoff, senior editor at Skyhorse, I am so grateful to you for believing in me as a first-time author and giving me a chance to share my story and hopefully inspire others.

To my editor, Andres Dietz-Chavez at Skyhorse, thank you so much for your input and your guidance.

And to Herta Feely, my editor from Chrysalis Editorial, I am forever grateful to you for your patience, your insight, and for guiding me through a year of rewrites. Your immediate connection with me through being a mom of two athletic and adventurous boys was without a doubt a reason for our instant friendship.

Of course I have to thank the coaches and mentors in my life, Tracy Sundlun, Hank Lange, Troy Jacobson and the gang at Runners Edge in Farmingdale, New York, and the Falls Road Running Group in Baltimore, Maryland, for pushing me and helping me reach my potential as an athlete and ultimately discover my passion and the life lessons that proved so valuable.